Food Hygiene for Caterers

Food Hygiene for Caterers

GAYNOR CURTIS

ROBERT HALE · LONDON

First published in Great Britain 1993

ISBN 0 7090 5262 6

Robert Hale Limited
Clerkenwell House
Clerkenwell Green
London EC1R 0HT

Photoset in Times by
Derek Doyle & Associates, Mold, Clwyd.
Printed in Great Britain by
St Edmundsbury Press Ltd, Bury St Edmunds, Suffolk.
Bound by WBC Bookbinders Ltd, Bridgend, Mid-Glamorgan.

Contents

Introduction

Food is vital to enable people to live and thrive, but if the food they eat is contaminated it can cause illness or even death.

The number of cases of food poisoning reported in Great Britain is increasing, and many people are suffering unpleasant illnesses. Some vulnerable members of society, for example, the very young, the sick and the elderly, are at risk of dying should they suffer the symptoms of food poisoning.

Caterers should aim to prevent food poisoning ever happening. It can be prevented as easily as it is caused. If all food handlers were aware of the problems they can cause when they handle, store or prepare food incorrectly, there would be less cases of food poisoning. This book is intended to inform caterers of every aspect of current hygiene rules and regulations. It will enable the caterer to counter, answer and deal with any problem that may crop up.

The Food Safety Act 1990 has been introduced to control the standards of food offered for sale, and the preparation and service of food. It affects everyone working in catering, and is designed to protect the consumer from eating contaminated food. It is important to understand the Act's implications for a catering business. A shop or restaurant may have been running for many years with no problems or cases of food poisoning. On the whole, any clean and well-run kitchen will not pose a problem, but there are rising cases of bacterial food poisoning.

Everyone who handles food needs to know how to prevent customers from becoming ill or dying, and they need to know the latest hygiene requirements. Food poisoning does not happen as an oversight in one department or as a result of one mistake. There is no proof that a cobweb or a cracked tile in the kitchen means that premises cannot consistently produce safe food. Food poisoning happens because of a series of events. Bacteria have to get into the food in the first place and then have the conditions necessary for them to grow and multiply.

The general public are becoming more aware of food hygiene and cleanliness of premises. Businesses that take this legislation seriously, and attempt to comply with it, may achieve higher sales through increased customer confidence, loyalty and satisfaction.

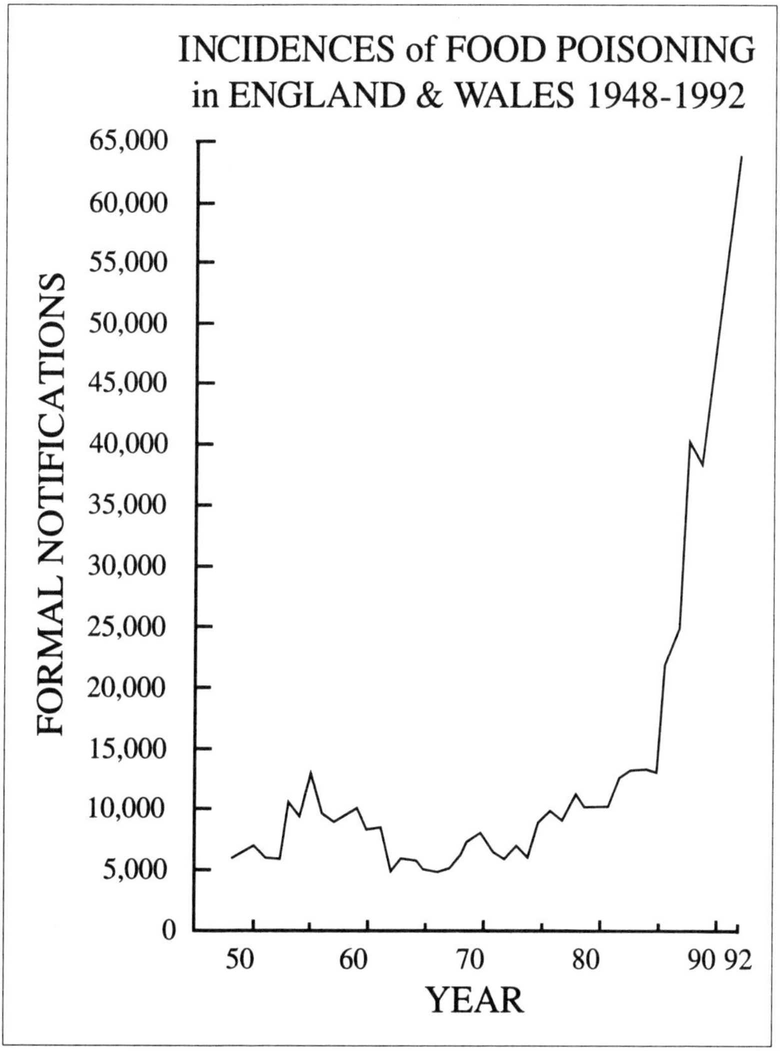
INCIDENCES of FOOD POISONING
in ENGLAND & WALES 1948-1992
FORMAL NOTIFICATIONS
65,000
60,000
55,000
50,000
45,000
40,000
35,000
30,000
25,000
20,000
15,000
10,000
5,000
0
50
60
70
80
90 92
YEAR

1 Premises and Equipment

KITCHEN LAYOUT

The correct layout of equipment in food premises is of great importance to the maintenance of a high standard of cleanliness. The size, shape and purpose of food premises varies considerably, but there are certain general principles which will maintain a high standard of cleanliness and avoid contamination of food.

The greater the distance food has to be carried and the more often it is handled, the greater the chance of the food becoming contaminated. It is important that equipment should be planned in a forward-moving manner.

This principle applies to all kitchens, cafeterias, shops etc. Vegetable storage and preparation should be near to the delivery door and not carried through the kitchen. Dust and soil on the vegetables may settle on other foods.

In siting equipment, the fullest use should be made of natural light and consideration should be given to artificial lighting so that there are no dark corners, passages etc. to collect unseen dirt and so that dirt and spillages are evident and can be cleaned immediately.

Machinery and large equipment should be sited so that it and the surrounding walls and floors can be easily cleaned.

Narrow spaces are difficult to clean and tend to provide areas where food and insects can lodge.

Don't put two large pieces of equipment back to back. The tendency will be not to move them apart for cleaning. If the items are electrical you will need to ensure the motors are not touching and there are no cables or wires trailing the floor to reach the equipment. If they are large items used for frying or grilling, extraction would be needed above them.

The central island layout is ideal for food preparation but keep the large pieces of equipment used for refrigeration and cooking against a wall. This makes it easier to pull out and clean behind and extraction is easier to site on walls.

Work tables and benches should be movable to ease floor cleaning. If equipment stands on legs, the legs must be long enough to allow for thorough cleaning underneath and to allow the floor to be easily inspected.

All unit cupboards, benches, etc. should be completely sealed against dirt penetration, and these units should be placed so that they can be cleaned on all sides.

Refrigerators should be placed away from heated areas so that they can work efficiently.

LIGHTING

It is essential that all food preparation areas are sufficiently and adequately lighted. Arrangements for high-level cleaning of the lights must be made. Lighting should be bright enough to prevent accidents and shadow free (e.g. neon), so that dirt is readily visible and the kitchen can be cleaned thoroughly.

WALLS

The walls of any food area should have a smooth surface, which is easy to clean, and be of a light colour so that dirt is easily visible. Ceramic tiles make a good long-term investment when the cost and time of painting the walls is considered. They should be cleaned regularly, even at high levels, and cleaned with a cloth using a proprietary cleaner. A sterilizer should be used behind sinks and walls where splashes of food may occur. The space behind false walls must be sealed to prevent access to insects and pests.

CEILINGS

Ceilings in the food preparation area should have a smooth finish to facilitate cleaning. The finish should be smooth, jointless, impervious to grease and moisture, light in colour and fire-resistant. Solid or fibre board ceilings should be coved where they meet the edges. An absorbent plaster painted with a washable emulsion is suitable, but gloss paint should not be used as this increases condensation. Polystyrene tiles are unsuitable because of the fire risk and because they are difficult to clean. Ceilings should be cleaned regularly.

FLOORS

A kitchen floor must be made of a hardwearing, easy to clean, anti-slip and non-absorbent material. It should be resistant to acids, fats or grease. It should have no breaks or cracks and crevices as these provide good sites for dirt and bacteria to accumulate.

Satisfactory Flooring Materials
Ideally floors should be made from thick, non-slip vinyl sheets. The flooring should meet the walls with coving to prevent bacteria and pests from moving in under the skirting-boards. Quarry tiles with an abrasive finish to prevent slipping are suitable. They withstand wear, chemicals, heat and are vermin proof. Terrazzo is satisfactory if used on smaller areas; on larger areas it tends to crack and can be a little slippery.

Unsatisfactory Flooring Materials
Wood block is unsuitable for kitchens and food preparation rooms since food waste and insects may lodge in the joins and it can be slippery. Concrete is very dusty, particularly when sweeping operations are in progress. Rubber is also unsuitable as it is slippery when fat and water are present. Asphalt (composition) softens in heat and under the weight of heavy machinery, sugars and fats act on its surface to produce ‘pitting’, which renders the floor difficult to clean. Timber is very unsatisfactory. It is absorbent and easily

stained, dust accumulates in the joints and it is not vermin proof. Timber should always be covered in an impervious material such as tiles or vinyl if it must be used.

Cleaning of Floors

An electric floor scrubber will thoroughly clean the floor area of large kitchens. A tankful of hot water and detergent suds are sucked up leaving a clean, dry floor. If you have a smaller area to clean, sweep it first (try to avoid raising dust), then use a mop and bucket with hot water and detergent or a proprietary cleaner, and rinse with clean water. Dispose of the resulting dirty water, rinse the bucket and disinfect the mop. Always walk backwards to avoid walking on areas that are already clean, but take care not to injure yourself or others. Warning cones or notices should be put out to warn others that the floor is being cleaned.

VENTILATION

Removal of Vapours and Fumes from Cooking and Processing

It is a requirement of the Food Hygiene Regulations that 'sufficient and suitable means of ventilation shall be provided in every food room and suitable and sufficient ventilation shall be maintained'.

This ventilation is necessary for:

The extraction of cooking fumes;
The prevention of condensation;
The provision of a healthy atmosphere for the staff;
The prevention of a hot, close, steamy atmosphere in which the growth of bacteria is greatly encouraged.

Ventilation problems vary according to the size, shape, height, layout and equipment of a kitchen, and also according to the number of staff in the kitchen and the demands on the establishment.

Ventilation may be obtained either naturally or mechanically.

Natural Ventilation

Natural ventilation is not very suitable since windows only provide ventilation in certain kinds of weather, even if the windows are properly sited and their opening can be adjusted according to the needs of the room. Windows need to be insectproof and fitted with screens.

Mechanical Ventilation

Mechanical ventilation is based on a combination of a canopy, ducting and fans exhausting the hot, damp and greasy air together with a controlled fresh air replacement system. Fumes and steam are removed immediately, as the canopy is fitted over all the cooking equipment.

Canopies must be made of easily cleaned material, stainless steel is best, and project at least 18″ on the sides, and they should be about 6′ 9″ from the floor. Canopies should not have any horizontal dust collecting surfaces, and they should be fitted with a small gutter around the bottom to collect up any condensed steam. Exhaust fans should be adjustable to give the necessary air changes in the kitchen without producing draughts.

Fresh air comes through doors, windows etc., and sometimes this air is heated by providing fresh air inlets placed behind radiators. Extraction is not efficient if there is not the right supply of fresh air. Mechanical ventilation can also be obtained by fitting an injector fan with a filter fitted at one end of the room and an extractor fan fitted at the other end.

If cooking and washing-up equipment is placed against an outer wall, fumes can be extracted naturally by the use of outlet vents. The outlet should be protected against the entry of foreign matter, and the flue should be extended to the top of the building, so that the fumes etc. are kept clear of the building.

CELLARS

Drink is classified as food and is subject to the Food Safety Act 1990 and the Food Hygiene Regulations 1970.

There are essential conditions and equipment vital for any

bar cellar. They include:

Good adequate lighting;
Cold water supply;
Stainless steel buckets;
Mallet for tapping casks;
Hard and soft spiles;
Washers for cask top connectors;
CO_2 bottle spanner;
Cask top spanner.

Any faults should be reported to the equipment suppliers immediately.

CLEANING

Insanitary Premises (Regulation 6, Food Hygiene (Amended) Regulations 1989)
A food business must not be carried on in any premises where the situation, condition or construction is such that food is exposed to the risk of contamination. Insanitary premises will include those infested with pests, with defective or leaking drains or where there is such a lack of cleaning that the premises are filthy. This also includes premises which are not easy to keep clean and hygienic because of poor structural condition.

A breach of this Food Hygiene Regulation is likely to result in the issue of an Emergency Prohibition Notice (Section 12).

The aim of cleaning is to remove visible waste food and dirt, and to destroy the bacteria that will be present in waste food and dirt. It is important to establish a routine of cleaning and to use the maxim 'CLEAN AS YOU GO'. The Food Hygiene Regulations (reg. 6 & reg. 7) has a legal requirement for the 'food premises to be kept clean and not pose a health risk'.

The definition of cleaning has been described as 'the application of energy using heat, chemicals and physical work to remove dirt and grease'.

All parts of the structure and the equipment within the

kitchen must be regularly cleaned. It must be part of the working day and become a priority job task. You must consider whether a piece of equipment, or a work surface that comes into contact with food, can cause direct or indirect contamination of otherwise clean food. It is vital that surfaces upon which food is prepared are kept clean and bacteria free.

CLEANING SCHEDULES

All areas of food premises must be cleaned on a regular basis. A cleaning routine should list the items to be cleaned and the staff allocated to the task. The cleaning schedule should identify the following:

The areas and equipment to be cleaned;
How often items need cleaning;
The required standard;
The equipment and methods necessary;
The chemicals to be used;
The person who will undertake the task, and the person who will supervise it;
The safety precautions necessary, together with the first-aid provision.

A cleaning schedule should be easy to understand, simple to follow and applicable to the premises. Make it relevant, devise a system which identifies areas often seen as being difficult to clean, include walls behind sinks, ovens, hot cupboards and low fixed shelves, areas inside dishwashers, between cookers, behind and under pipes, the sides of refrigerators and freezers and any immovable equipment. Other areas that should not be missed are the undersides of tables and the edges, the undersides of shelves, the inner seals of refrigerators, can openers, slicers, drains and gullies, all internal surfaces of machines, drawers, door handles, switches and cables.

These are areas commonly spotted by an Environmental Health Officer.

DO keep records of cleaning schedules for six months as they can be used to prove 'due diligence'.

DO monitor the cleaning system, check that cleaning is being carried out and that it is up to the required standards.

Examples of recent court cases that were brought because of poor cleaning standards are:

DIRTY PUB KITCHEN £2,000 FINE

Just four months after being totally refurbished, an EHO (Environmental Health Officer) found grease and food debris all over the kitchen walls and floors of the pub, and some parts of the kitchen were described as 'filthy'. The brewery was fined £2,000 with £150 costs for failing to keep kitchen walls and floors clean, failing to keep the kitchen ceiling in such a condition it could be cleaned and infestation prevented, failing to keep a washbasin clean and failing to keep articles and equipment clean, namely a steam cooker, potato peeler and gas cooker. The officer also found a hole in the ceiling and food debris on the walls, ceiling, washbasin and other equipment.

BAKERY FINED £900

Carrying on a business on insanitary premises. EHOs found dirty trays, dirty fridges, food waste under equipment and beetles in the flour.

RESTAURANT OWNER FINED £7,000 WITH £170 COSTS

The owner admitted seventeen charges under the Food Hygiene Regulations. The court was told the premises had been infested with rats for some time, and inspectors found a decomposed rat carcass under a food display cabinet, rat droppings on shelves, and the remains of a rat's nest. Grease deposits were found throughout the premises on walls, ceilings and equipment. Mouldy and inedible food was also found.

RESTAURANT OWNER FINED £3,200 WITH £777 COSTS

He admitted twenty charges, including accumulation of food waste, dirt and grease, potential for rodent and insect infestation, a cockroach under the refrigerator, a larder beetle and fly pupae in a food preparation room and storage room, rat droppings, food at risk from contamination during preparation, cooked food left out overnight and a long-term lack of cleaning.

CLEANING CHEMICALS

There is now an extensive range of products for cleaning available from a wide range of suppliers. No single cleaning product will be suitable for all cleaning jobs, there is no 'all purpose cleaner' for catering tasks, different chemicals are needed for different tasks. The products fall into four categories:

Detergent
Sterilizer
Sanitizer
Disinfectant

Detergents
Detergents are chemicals which act with water on a surface, even if it is greasy. They will clean by allowing the whole surface to become wet, and are designed to remove waste food, dirt and grease. Washing-up liquid is an example of a detergent: it does not kill bacteria, but will reduce the number present by removing the waste, dirt and grease that contain bacteria. Detergents are used simply to remove dirt from surfaces, equipment, crockery etc. They have no bacteriacidal properties and will not kill bacteria. Their function is to cut through and remove grease and dirt which may prevent sterilization of the article concerned. A good detergent should have the following properties:

Be non-poisonous and non-corrosive;
Be readily soluble in all types of water;
Have good wetting and suspending powers, to ensure adequate penetration of dirt, and to prevent a scum forming on the surface of the washing water;
Be able to break down fats and oils;
Have a good temperature range, i.e. be able to keep its penetrating and cleaning properties over a wide range of temperatures;
Be easily rinsed away.

Detergents are usually made from soap or a soap substitute manufactured as a by-product of the oil industry. Soap is the simplest type of detergent but its use for washing up is limited in hard water areas. Most good detergents incorporate a water softening agent such as common washing soda (sodium carbonate) or other salts of sodium. These help to keep the salts of hard water in solution so that the cleaning agent is more effective.

DO NOT allow staff to mix washing-up liquid with any other cleaning chemical.

Sterilizers

Sterilizers are chemicals which kill bacteria and spores present on surfaces and equipment, but will not remove waste food and dirt alone; for this reason, a surface or equipment will have to be cleaned before a sterilizer is applied. Steam is a sterilizer, so a dishwasher using a detergent to wash and then boiling water to rinse, will sterilize. A good sterilizer should have the following properties:

Be non-poisonous and non-corrosive;
Be soluble in water;
Have high germicidal efficiency;
Have a good temperature range;
Be non-tainting;
Have a Rideal Walker co-efficient of four or over. (The Rideal Walker co-efficient is a test used to compare the 'killing power' of a particular sterilant with that of a standard concentration of Phenol.)

There is no official recommendation governing sterilants for use in the kitchen, but those recommended for use in the dairy industry by the Milk and Dairies (General) Regulations 1959 are suitable. These are split down into several groups, the most popular being:

Sodium Hypochlorite solutions, which include Delsanex, Domestos, Chlosan, and Quaternary Ammonium Compounds (QUATS) which include BHC, Sterex, Lactosan;

Sterilants based on available chlorine, which include Bactron, Circlor, Atlasan.

These types are of a dual nature and are known as detergents/sterilizers. They combine the properties and make it unnecessary to use separate chemicals in the cleaning routine. Remember that the safest method for destroying bacteria is HEAT, which is a sterilizing technique.

Sanitizers

Sanitizers are chemicals which are both detergents and sterilizers; they will remove waste food, dirt and grease and kill bacteria. There are products commercially available for washing up and cleaning surfaces. Chemical disinfectants can be inactivated by dirt and food residues, so choose your products carefully. A detergent wash followed by a sterilizer is more effective than a sanitizer on dirty equipment and surfaces.

Disinfectants

Disinfectants are chemicals capable of destroying bacteria; spores will survive disinfection, but disinfecting articles after washing with detergent will prevent food poisoning occuring from bacteria present on equipment. Disinfectants have no cleaning properties and are useless as a detergent. Their function is to kill any bacteria left after the detergent has cleaned the surface in question. Very few disinfectants are suitable for use on food contact surfaces because most of them will taint food. They may leave a strong taste or smell on the surface, they (particularly bleach) can leave a toxic residue behind and they can discolour surfaces. Many excellent disinfectants are suitable for use outside the kitchen to disinfect toilets, drains, walls, waste bins etc. Three types of disinfectants are used in the food industry.

Sodium Hypochlorite (e.g. bleach) was used extensively as a disinfectant until quite recently. It is cheap, removes stains and kills bacteria and viruses. Common household bleach is the most effective disinfectant available, but there is much disagreement over the suitability of its use in a food environment. Some city councils have banned the use of bleach for any purpose from all their premises, including school canteens, office kitchens etc. Hypochlorite bleach when mixed with an acid preparation produces chlorine (which can seriously damage the lungs). A hypochlorite bleach mixed with a liquid cleaner with ammonium compounds produces acid fumes. Any mixing of acid products with alkali creates heat, and the reaction can be violent enough to spray corrosive liquid in all directions.

Iodophors, which are complexes of detergents and iodine, kill a wide range of micro-organisms, but they attack some metals and are expensive.

QACs (QUATs) are cationic detergents (e.g. Savlon) and are suitable for use on both steel and plastic surfaces, but they are not fast acting and do not kill bacterial spores. They are inactivated in the presence of organic matter (food!) and are expensive when compared with hypochlorites.

You should follow certain rules when handling cleaning chemicals:

FOLLOW THE MANUFACTURER'S INSTRUCTIONS
Containers that have been decanted from a large container should have a clearly written label stating the instruction for use. Always follow such instructions as 'use gloves' or 'wear goggles' or 'wear a mask'!

DO NOT USE AT A GREATER STRENGTH THAN SPECIFIED
This is wasteful, literally pouring money down the drain. The quantities that the manufacturer recommends are the right quantities for the job. Increasing the strength does not mean it will do the job any better.

NEVER MIX CHEMICALS
Mixing chemicals is a really dangerous practice. For example, there is the all too common practice of mixing washing-up liquid with bleach to mop the floor. Some people have said that they 'swear by it, it really does the job well'. This is a very flawed reasoning:

a) it negates the cleaning power of the detergent;
b) it deactivates the germicide in the bleach;
c) it causes a chemical reaction;
d) it will wear out the mop head quickly.

Mixing detergents with any other chemical should be positively discouraged; mixing detergent with an acid household cleaner produces a potentially lethal chloric gas.

At the other end of the scale, the following report was made recently:

In a bid to unblock the toilet at their home, the husband put sulphuric acid down the toilet. He told his wife not to put anything else down there, but after four days of flushing she thought it would be safe. She put bleach down the pan and immediately the pan began to bubble, creating deadly gases which filtered through the house. Minutes later as she and her husband began to feel nauseous and dizzy, they called the fire service. The house was evacuated, the fumes filtered out into the street and three firemen waiting outside were hit by the gas and had to be taken to hospital. Other firemen, wearing breathing apparatus, dismantled the toilet to reach the drains.

The couple had created a deadly chlorine cocktail in their bid to unblock the toilet by the mixing of two chemicals. The husband's final comment was 'it's awful to think what would have happened if we had gone to bed. We might not be here today.'

NEVER mix chemicals.

STORE CHEMICALS SAFELY AWAY FROM FOOD

Chemicals should be stored in a clearly marked cupboard that states CLEANING AGENTS ONLY. This ensures there is no risk that chemicals will be accidently mixed if boxes split or containers are knocked over and come into contact with food.

DO NOT store chemicals under the sink. This is probably the dampest place in the food handling area, cartons will deteriorate and chemicals can leak out. For safety reasons, and to comply with COSHH regulations, technical information on a data sheet must be provided by the supplier of each chemical supplied. The data sheet should include the following information:

A list of chemical compounds;
The working exposure limits for each component;
The details of any known human reaction with other substances;
The recommended precautions for handling and storage;
The recommended precautions in the event of emergencies (fire, spillages);
The results of any relevant tests (flammable? explosive? toxic?);
Any hazards indicated by research or experience of use ;
Information on the measured levels of exposure for the person using the product.

DO ensure that the supplied information on safety and handling covers these points.

Broadly speaking, any chemical may produce a toxin or irritant effect if it comes into contact with the skin; if it is breathed in in the form of dusts, gases, vapours or spray aerosols; or through ingestion or contact with the eyes.

DO wear protective gloves and/or barrier cream when handling chemicals.
DO wash hands after handling chemicals and before eating, smoking or drinking.
DO wear goggles when handling liquid chemicals to protect the eyes from accidental splashing.
DO check the directions for use, and ensure adequate ventilation when using chemicals by spray.

WASHING UP

By Hand

Scrape off any waste food then pre-rinse. Add detergent to the water to help remove waste food and dirt. The temperature of the water should be around 50°C. This is too hot for bare hands so rubber gloves should be worn. The items should be scrubbed with a tough nylon bristle brush to remove any visible waste food and dirt. Then rinse the items with very hot water around 70-80°C to rinse off any remnants of detergent and kill bacteria. The high temperature of the water will ensure that the items will be hot and air dry. Wherever possible allow equipment to air dry. If a wipe has to be used to dry the equipment, use disposable paper products. There is no need to use a tea-towel or drying cloth.

Wiping-down cloths have been identified time and time again as a means of cross contamination when a cloth is used first to wipe an infected surface and then to wipe equipment used for cooked food.

An example of cross contamination:

A widespread outbreak of salmonella poisoning in 1947 included 3,000-4,000 cases resulting in three deaths. An infected pig carcass contaminated other carcasses in the slaughterhouse when wiping-down cloths were used. This raw meat was distributed to butcher shops and handled with cooked meats. The infective raw meat and the cooked cold meats were weighed on the same scale, cut with the same knife and handled with the same hands.

The point of this story is that cross contamination is prevented not just by separating storage areas, equipment and working surfaces, or cleaning and sterilizing after use, but by the cloth used for wiping down. There is little or no argument for using cloths. The range of disposable products is now so extensive, and relatively cheap, that the costs far outweigh the costs of food poisoning. Cloths are used for long periods, they harbour bacteria and cause cross contamination.

DO use, wherever possible, paper or sanitizing wipes.
DO use once then throw them away. If this is not possible or practical, purchase a wipe made of short-lived material and dispose of it at the end of the service period.
DO NOT leave wipes in warm water at the sides of the sinks. Rinse them after use and leave to dry out.

Washing by Machine
There are many different makes and types of dishwashers on the market, and they all follow the same stages of cleaning described in 'Washing by hand', i.e. equipment is washed in hot water and detergent, then rinsed and disinfected with

hot water sprays or steam.

DO ensure the hot water reaches a temperature of 49-60°C.
DO check the rinsing water is between 66-80°C. Steam can be used to disinfect.
DO ensure the machine is correctly and neatly loaded so that the detergent and hot water can reach every item.
DO check regularly that the machine is working properly and that the correct temperatures are being maintained. A machine that is not working properly is a hazard.

Pot Washing
Pots should be washed separately from other crockery and cutlery. Follow the guidelines for washing by hand or machine. Scourers made from stainless steel or steel, whilst very effective for scouring and restoring a shine to aluminium utensils, can loose bits of the metal fibres and eventually end up in the food. Abrasive pads made from plastic fibres are good, but these can be damaging to aluminium surfaces and should be used in accordance with the manufacturer's instructions.

EQUIPMENT

Articles or equipment used for the preparation or storage of food must be kept clean and in good condition. They should be made of a non-porous material. Equipment such as ovens, refrigerators, freezers and tables should be movable to promote effective cleaning of the equipment. There is a risk of cross contamination with equipment that is used for both raw and cooked foods e.g. chopping-boards, slicers and knives, and, where possible, the same equipment should not be used for both without sanitizing between use.

When purchasing equipment consideration should be given to:

The design;
The materials from which it is made;
The construction and working.

Thus it can be assessed whether or not the equipment can be cleaned thoroughly by a person of ordinary intelligence and mechanical ability. No piece of equipment should cause the person cleaning it to neglect the operation because it is too complicated in design or construction.

Design of Equipment

The most satisfactory design is that which has the greatest area of smooth unbroken surfaces. There should be:

No ornamentation;
No unnecessary ridges, projections etc.;
No internal corners;
No dust traps.

Equipment with plain, smooth surfaces can be easily cleaned and readily examined to make sure it is clean.

Materials from which Equipment is Made

These materials should ensure that the food with which it comes into contact is not contaminated. Generally speaking, the materials should be:

Hard;
Smooth;
Non-absorbent;
Resistant to rust;
Resistant to chipping.

The types of materials in common use are:

Aluminium: Cast or wrought aluminium is not very hard and does not resist scratches. Should not be used with acid foods.
Copper: This is hard-wearing, strong and reasonably hard, but it corrodes easily to form a poisonous film (verdegris). The inside of utensils etc. should be lined with tin.
Enamel: This chips or splinters as the result of hard blows or excessive heat. It should never be used for acidic liquids.
Galvanized Zinc: This is liable to corrode, and if acid foods are mixed in zinc containers zinc in poisonous quantities may be absorbed into food.

Glass: Toughened glass is not to be recommended in the light of possible breakage and cost.
Marble: This is a good hard surface, easily cleaned. Ideal surface for fats and pastry.
Plastics: These are light, splinter-proof, reasonably impervious, pliable and less breakable than glass or china.
Stainless Steel: Ideal material for most purposes. Does not easily corrode, withstands food and cleaning chemicals, suffers no damage from reasonable heating, freezing and does not chip or crack.
Tinned Equipment: This is satisfactory when tinning is adequate, but the tinned surface can be removed by heat or through wear exposing the base metal.
Wood: Is generally undesirable because it is absorbent and cannot be thoroughly cleaned. Soft wood is most unsatisfactory as it will absorb moisture, is easily scratched and cut, cannot be easily cleaned and so allows the multiplication of food poisoning bacteria. Hard wood can be used for butcher's chopping-blocks because the surface can be ground down when showing signs of wear.

CHOPPING-BOARDS

Under the Food Hygiene Regulations a chopping-board is classed as: 'an article of equipment that is likely to come into contact with food, therefore it has to be kept clean, made of a material that enables it to be kept clean, in good order, repair and condition, and to prevent any matter being absorbed by the board. It should not present any risk of contamination to the food'. Regulation 6 also states: 'that in determining whether any item is clean, regard should be made to the nature and packing of the food for which the item is required, and to the use made by the item'. This means that the standards of cleanliness needed for chopping raw meat, for example, will differ from slicing bread, because bread will not need any further preparation before being eaten. Chopping-boards are work surfaces and used in all stages of food preparation for cutting, chopping and slicing. The reason a chopping-board is used is that a stainless steel surface or a formica surface could damage the knives being used, or the work surface itself. The surface of the board should be:

Firm enough to take the work being done;
Non-slip;
Hygienic and easy to clean;
Undamaged and unable to harbour bacteria.

For many years the only chopping-boards used were made of wood, wood being cheap and durable. Now wood is considered unsuitable and unacceptable for safe food hygiene. With prolonged use the wood gets scratched, and moisture penetrates the softer wood underneath. Bacteria can then survive and multiply inside the board. If the surface becomes scratched and pitted or even split, the board can no longer be thoroughly cleaned and sanitized, and should be replaced. Modern materials such as polypropylene have been developed, and are ideal for use as chopping-boards. They are non-absorbent, long-lasting and easy to clean. However, they too will eventually become worn, scrached or damaged and should be replaced when necessary. They are widely available, with a colour coding system that enables the food handler to select the correct board for the job in hand, so reducing the risk of cross contamination. These boards are made of material that can be washed, sanitized, disinfected or sterilized in very hot water. You can select your own method of colour coding, for example:

RED	Raw meat only
YELLOW	Raw poultry only
GREEN	Salad preparation only
BROWN	Cooked meats only
BLACK	Dairy products only
BLUE	Raw fish only

Knives can also be marked in the same way to cut down the risk of cross contamination.

REFRIGERATORS

As temperatures fall, bacterial activity declines, therefore foods which support bacterial growth should be stored at low temperatures. The refrigerator usually operates at a temperature between 1° and 5°C and can be used for the short-term storage of various foods. This will normally prevent the growth of pathogens, but many spoilage bacteria will continue to grow at refrigeration temperatures of around 4°C, thus spoilage can occur even within the refrigerator. Once food is removed from the refrigerator, bacterial growth is resumed. The function of a refrigerator is to keep food cool, not normally, to cool hot food. Hot food will raise the temperature of the refrigerator, causing all the food stored in it to come into the 'danger zone', the atmosphere becomes saturated with water and further problems arise.

DO NOT store foods that are decomposing.
DO NOT store foods that are strong-smelling or may contaminate by odour any other foods (unless kept in an airtight container).
DO NOT store foods which need to be kept dry and well ventilated.
DO NOT store cans and bottles, unless specified and unless there is sufficient space. Priority must be given to meat, cream, milk, custards and gravy.
DO NOT store frozen foods unless they are being defrosted.
DO NOT allow the refrigerator to become overcrowded. If this happens there may be insufficient ventilation to keep the food-stuffs in proper condition although the food may be cool.
DO enable air to circulate freely.
DO place liquids close to the freezing coils, meat products further away, eggs and other products furthest away.
DO store raw meat and poultry at the bottom of the refrigerator.
DO inspect the refrigerator daily and check stocks of stored food to make sure everything is in good condition.
DO throw away any decomposing foods.

CHILL ROOMS

Chill rooms are used in larger catering establishments to store foods which will deteriorate at room temperature. They operate as an ordinary refrigerator with temperatures between 0° and 4°C, depending on the type of food needing storage. Designed and used correctly they will allow food to be cooled more quickly and safely than at room temperature.

Consideration must be given to the following points. It should have been specifically designed as a chill room. It must have sufficient refrigeration capacity to extract the increased heat load. The cooling of foods must not increase the storage temperature of other foods in the chill room. Shelving must be solid, lightweight and allow easy cleaning. Open mesh shelving will allow air to circulate better, cooling food more quickly. Chill rooms must be cleaned regularly with a mild odourless cleaner.

FREEZERS

The length of time that food can be safely stored in a freezer depends on the temperature of the freezer. The star marking system indicates the temperature of the freezer and the length of time that the products can be stored.

	Temperature of Freezer	Food storage time
★	–6°C	1 week
★★	–12°C	1 month
★★★	–18°C	3 months
★★★★	–18 to –25°C	3 months or longer and capable of freezing fresh food

Bacteria will not be killed at freezer temperatures but remain dormant until conditions are ideal for growth. Food that has been frozen tends to allow more rapid bacterial growth than the equivalent fresh foods.

DO NOT re-freeze frozen food which has started to defrost.

In an ice-cream freezer (conservator):

DO NOT store anything but ice-cream in the cabinet.
DO keep cabinet lids in position.

DO keep lids on individual containers of ice cream.
DO maintain lids in good condition or the temperature will rise and the ice cream deteriorate.
DO defrost and clean at regular intervals.

MICROWAVES

Cooking and reheating foods in a microwave is now a common cooking method used in many establishments. Microwave cooking differs from conventional cooking. In conventional cooking, heat is applied to the food from an outside heat source. In microwave cooking, microwaves act on the molecules in the food, particularly the water molecules, causing them to move against each other causing friction and creating heat which spreads inwards through the food by conduction. Microwaves penetrate the food to a depth of 3-5 cms, so that smaller portions of food will heat up and cook more quickly than larger ones. It is a fallacy that 'microwaves heat food from the inside to the outside', the outside edges of the food will always receive the most heat. The chief use of microwaves in a catering kitchen is in quickly reheating pre-cooked foods and thus eliminating the need for the food to be kept hot for long periods. Food cooked in a microwave, due to the reduction in time, will not go brown or crisp, and nutritional losses (i.e. the destruction of Vitamin C) are very similar to the losses in conventional oven cooking.

Caterers should use commercially designed microwave ovens, not domestic-type ovens. Commercial ovens are more robust, have a larger capacity and operate on a higher power setting, thus reducing the cooking time. Domestic ovens (usually around 650 watts) will reheat 12 oz of chilli con carne in 6 minutes, whereas a commercial oven (at 1,200 watts) will reheat it in 1½ minutes.

Equipment Used in a Microwave
Ceramics: See chinaware.
Chinaware: Check to see that it is marked 'microwave safe'. Some china will feel hot when removed from the microwave. This means it is absorbing microwave energy and, although safe to use, it will increase cooking/reheating times.

Cling film: Both PVC cling film and PVDC 'microwave' cling film are safe to use provided they do not come into contact with food. PVC has a lower temperature tolerance than PVDC, PVC softens at 130°C rather than 150°C. Government recommendations are that PVC can be used for defrosting or reheating food. When cooking in a microwave it can be used for covering containers, but not as a lining or in contact with food.
Earthenware: This is suitable, but thick containers will absorb some microwave energy away from the food and lead to increased cooking/reheating times.
Paper: Disposable polyester napkins, plates and cups are all suitable.
Plastics: Use rigid rather than soft plastics. Soft plastics such as reusable margarine tubs have not been designed for use in a microwave. The constituents could leak into the food at high temperatures and it will feel hot.
Porcelain: See chinaware.
Toughened glass: See chinaware.

DO NOT use metal or foil in a microwave. They reflect microwave energy and can damage the oven. China etc. with a metallic pattern should not be used in a microwave unless marked 'microwave safe'.

When cooking or reheating there are certain factors that affect the process, and they all depend on the wattage of the oven:

Refrigerated food will need a longer reheating time than food at room temperature;
If you double the portions of food to be reheated, reheating times increase by 50-75%;
Non-stirrable foods, such as shepherd's pie, need a longer heating time than sauces or vegetables, but will need a shorter standing time;
Foods high in sugar, salt or fat need a shorter reheating time than foods high in starchy carbohydrates or protein;
The shape of the container used for reheating is important. Round dishes are better than square ones. The corners of square dishes receive more microwave energy which could

lead to the corners of the food being overcooked whilst the centre remains cold. Shallow dishes will reheat food faster than deep dishes. Earthenware and china will slow down the heating process by absorbing the energy away from the food itself. Using a lid of any description means that the steam produced inside the container will fractionally reduce reheating times.

All foods reheated in a microwave should reach a centre temperature of 75°C to destroy listeria and salmonella bacteria. Suggested cooking and reheating times by the maker of the oven should be checked by temperature probing all foods, and a chart should be kept with proven reheating times. Amongst manufacturers of microwaves there is no standard language of power levels.

High	=	100% power
Medium High	=	70% power
Medium	=	50% power
Medium Low	=	30% power
Low	=	10% power

OR anything in between!

You need to run a physical check on power levels to reheat different foods. Draw up a chart that can be positioned at the microwave so that all users can check the times that different products need. Spend some time experimenting with the foods that are regularly reheated, e.g. roast chicken portions, steak pies etc. Take the product from the refrigerator, place in the microwave and set at two minutes on high. Remove the product and insert a temperature probe in the thickest part of the food. If the internal temperature reaches 70-75°C it is piping hot; if it has not reached this temperature return the product to the microwave for thirty seconds and check again. Continue until the correct temperature for the food is reached. Mark the product, the timing and the temperature on the chart and then throw away the product, as you have probed the food and cannot reheat it again.

Portion	Setting	Time	Final Temperature
Chicken Leg	High	2 mins	75°C
Steak pie	High	1½ mins	73°C

DO always stir the food halfway through cooking time and again before serving.
DO arrange the food. When reheating uneven pieces of food, put the thick part of one piece against the thin part of another, e.g. meaty piece of one chicken leg against the bony end of the other.
DO use a deep jug or bowl when reheating liquids, and check visually that the liquid is boiling.
DO make the potato mix in potato topped pies moister, and make sure the filling is deeper than the potatoes.
DO follow these rules for plated meals, the thinnest food in the centre, e.g. meat, dense food to the edges, e.g. potatoes. Cover where possible to trap steam.
DO NOT stack plates more than two high.

TOILETS

Sanitary conveniences situated in or regularly used by any food handler must be kept clean and well maintained. They should be positioned so that no offensive odour can penetrate into any food room. The room containing the toilet must be kept clean and properly lit and ventilated. No food, articles, or equipment likely to come into contact with food may be kept in any room containing a sanitary convenience. No food room which connects directly with a room containing a sanitary convenience can be used for the handling of open food.

Under the Health and Safety at Work Act 1974 there must be an intervening ventilated space between any room containing a sanitary convenience and a food room.

A clearly legible notice requesting food handlers to wash their hands must be fixed in a prominent position near every toilet used by them.

WASHHAND BASINS

All food premises must have a suitable and sufficient numbers of washhand basins for the use of food handlers, placed in the premises and in conveniently accessible positions (in close proximity to toilets, food preparation areas etc.) An adequate supply of hot and cold water, or hot water at a suitably controlled temperature should be provided. There must be liquid soap or suitable detergent available in a dispenser, and the type of soap chosen should be suitable for the water in the district. Nail-brushes must be supplied, preferably a nylon bristle-backed brush. The bristles should not be too harsh since these could damage the skin and increase the risk of infection. Nail-brushes must be kept at the washhand basin at all times, be readily available and visible. Suitable drying facilities must be available at each washhand basin. Communal roller towels are undesirable since they present a serious danger in transferring bacteria. Washhand basins must only be used for food handlers to wash their hands.

DO ensure that the washhand basin is always accessible.
DO keep it clean, and make sure that it is not used for anything else.
DO NOT put equipment in front of it so that it cannot be used.

FIRST-AID KIT

At least one first-aid kit should be provided to comply with the Food Safety Act 1990, which states 'it should be readily available and accessible. The contents should be adequate for the size of the business'. The kit should contain waterproof dressings of a distinctive colour. The Health and Safety at Work Act 1979 for food production premises requires the first-aid requirements that are listed in chapter 6 (see p. 174).

DO record any injury sustained by an employee which requires hospital treatment.
DO keep an accident book, regardless of the number of employees.

DO NOT keep pain-killing tablets on the premises. There was an incident where a young girl took a large number of tablets before going to work. She then asked her supervisor for two tablets for a headache. Those two tablets gave the girl an overdose.

DO NOT keep fabric plasters on the premises. (They pick up dirt easily.)

DO NOT keep antiseptic liquids. (Misuse in inexperienced hands.)

DO NOT keep burn sprays or creams in your first aid box. (If used incorrectly, blistering and scarring will not be prevented. Cold running water is the best initial treatment.)

2 Food

FOOD POISONING

Food poisoning is an illness brought about by eating food containing harmful substances or organisms. Unfit foods include mouldy foods, decomposing food and food containing food poisoning organisms or excessive additives. Contaminated food includes that containing foreign bodies, insect or rodent droppings. The main symptoms of food poisoning are diarrhoea, vomiting and abdominal pains. Vomiting and diarrhoea are the body's way of disposing of harmful substances from the digestive tract to prevent them from entering the blood stream. In a few types of food poisoning, the poison enters the blood stream causing illness with a wide variety of symptoms. The type of symptom and the time between eating the contaminated food and the start of the symptoms (incubation period) often helps to identify the type of food poisoning.

Food poisoning can affect people in two ways. The bacteria may enter the body in the food that is eaten, then cause a reaction either by invading the tissues of the intestine or by producing waste products that are poisonous. The bacteria can produce poisons (toxins) in the food itself, and when the food is eaten so are the poisons. Some bacteria do both (bacillus) and there is always the risk of eating poisons on or in food that is nothing to do with bacteria but is chemical in origin, e.g. pesticides on plants or cleaning powders in flour.

There are four types of food poisoning: chemical, poisonous plants, fungus and bacteria.

DO remember that bacteria are the main cause of food poisoning in Great Britain today.

Costs of Food Poisoning

Besides the fact that a customer is ill or has even died through eating infected food, there are other material costs to a business.

Loss of business. Reported food poisoning outbreaks means customer confidence and loyalty desert the business. Nobody will buy the product and money will be lost. Staff will be laid off and the reputation of the business suffers.

Renovation and replacing the equipment. The cost of commercial cleaning, renovating, repairing equipment and replacing equipment is a major capital expense. Can any business stand it?

Increased insurance premiums. Premiums will rise, the affected person may well demand and get compensation and public liability insurance will rise.

Legal action. The owner can be prosecuted, fined and/or imprisoned and disqualified from running a food business. The business can be closed down.

Increased salary costs. Staff may have to be replaced or more staff taken on.

Deaths

All types of food poisoning are life-threatening to certain members of the population. These groups are called high-risk groups and include the very young, the sick and the infirm, especially hospital patients, and the elderly. They are at risk of dying should they suffer the symptoms of food poisoning and the dehydration that comes with sickness and/or diarrhoea.

Dehydration is an abnormal loss of fluid from the body. Although people can go without food for several weeks without permanent harm, they can survive only a day or two without water. Dehydration occurs when people take in less fluid than they lose in urine, exhaled breath, perspiration, and faeces. Dehydration often accompanies excessive urination, vomiting and diarrhoea or loss of blood. Fever also causes water loss. With the high risk groups, dehydration is the most severe symptom of food poisoning and they are at risk of dying. With dehydration thirst is extreme, the mouth is dry and the skin is doughy and unresilient. The urine is dark, the patient becomes lethargic and nausea may develop. Acidosis and uraemia can occur. Prolonged dehydration leads to wasting and loss of weight.

Treatment includes drinking plenty of fluids. Where severe dehydration occurs through food poisoning, a saline solution, blood plasma or whole blood may be injected. The very young, babies and children under two, can become seriously ill very quickly if they start to dehydrate. Any projectile vomiting after feeding should be treated seriously and immediate medical advice sought.

Sick and elderly people are at particular risk and particular attention should be paid to safe food preparation for hospital or institutionalized patients. Their resistence is low and the dehydration that results from vomiting and diarrhoea is a killer. Normal healthy adults will recover from the effects of food poisoning quite quickly, but occasionally they too can become very ill and even die if the amount of bacteria present in the food is in large numbers.

In 1987 an elderly married couple, the wife aged sixty-five, the husband aged sixty-seven, bought ham, a pork pie and haslet from a local corner shop. Neither had eaten breakfast. The husband ate the pork pie and his wife had the ham. Later that day the couple were ill with diarrhoea, and the doctor confined them both to bed suspecting food poisoning. Two days later the husband felt better, but his wife's condition worsened and she was admitted to hospital. She died five days later. The inquest was told that she died from septicaemia shock caused by salmonella virchow and respiratory problems after the bacteria affected her lungs. It was discovered later that there were thirteen other reported cases of food poisoning on that day. All were traced to the same shop, but only this lady died.

All she did was buy and eat a slice of ham. She wasn't mugged or involved in a road accident – she bought food which killed her.

It is unsurprising that the Food Safety Act has been implemented to protect people and ensure their food is fit to eat.

The majority of reports of deaths from food poisoning involve persons over sixty. There is a greater risk if the person is both elderly and sick.

DO ensure strict standards of hygiene when handling baby bottles and equipment.

HIGH-RISK FOODS

These are foods which have consistently been identified as the source of a food poisoning outbreak. There are four types of high-risk foods: meat and poultry, milk and eggs, shellfish and seafood, cooked rice and all products made from them. These foods can be classified broadly into three groups:

1 Foods likely to be contaminated with large numbers of bacteria when they reach the kitchen. The stages of food preparation must kill the bacteria to prevent food spoilage or food poisoning. Examples include all meat and all poultry (some 80% of frozen chickens contain food poisoning bacteria) eggs and fish. Measure must be taken to prevent cross-contamination to other foods.
2 Foods which are safe but become high-risk, usually because of poor food handling, e.g. tinned meats, pasteurized milk or cream, custard, mayonnaise, milk powders, trifle mixes.
3 Foods already cooked and to be eaten cold, e.g. cold sliced cooked meats and savouries, cold sweets and cream-filled confectionary.

(Shellfish and seafood often feed in contaminated waters and cooked rice may contain the bacteria, bacillus cereus, which can survive the cooking process.)

Meat and Poultry
All meat and all poultry are now classed as high-risk food. High-risk foods are foods that have consistently been identified as having been the cause of an outbreak of food poisoning. Both salmonella and clostridium perfringens live in the intestines of animals and humans, the animals show no

symptoms and are just the carriers of the bacteria, so the bacteria can be transferred to meat intended for human consumption. Quality cuts of meat, e.g. sirloin, fillet, leg of lamb, are 'deep muscle' meats and are rarely a cause of food poisoning. If you or your customer have a preference for rare steak, this should not pose a problem since bacteria are mostly present on, or near, the surface of the meat. Steak should have been kept refrigerated and then be grilled quickly and served. Rolled joints and minced meat are often the cause of food poisoning because if the surface of the meat is contaminated the bacteria become rolled or minced throughout the meat. Bacteria will be present in the centre of a chicken, in the cavity from which the intestines have been removed. Thorough cooking of all poultry is necessary to kill the bacteria that will be present. Some meats, usually pork, are infected by worms, and some tapeworms affect fish. Trichinosis is a disease caused by infestation by a tiny roundworm called trichinella spiralis. It burrows into the intestinal wall and gives rise to enormous numbers of microscopic larvae, which then spread throughout the body by the lymph system of the bloodstream. Many such infections cause no symptoms; occasionally effects are very severe and may cause death. The usual symptoms are abdominal pain, muscular pain, swelling of the eyelids and pain around the eyes. The disease is transmitted by infected meat, usually pork. Cysts settle in the muscle of the infected animal. If the meat is not cooked properly or eaten raw the cysts survive and will develop in the human body into small worms. It is common in the USA, but occurs only occasionally in Britain due to routine meat inspection, however this is not a complete safeguard as cysts are difficult to detect.

DO cook pork thoroughly. This will kill any cysts. Trichinellae are destroyed if all parts of the meat reach a minimum of 60°C.
DO NOT store frozen pork above –20°C.

BSE: Bovine Spongiform Encephalopathy
BSE is a disease of cows caused by a micro-organism similar to a virus. The disease attacks the cow's brain and spinal

cord causing a progressive deterioration of the cow's central nervous system and finally death.

It is believed the disease resulted from manufacturers of cattle feed recycling animal carcasses to increase the protein content of the feed. Sheep have always been susceptible to a brain disease called scrapie and the use of sheep carcasses in the manufacture of cattle feed infected the feed, thus cows being fed the infected feed contracted this disease. The practice of incorporating animal carcasses into cattle feed is now prohibited under the BSE Order 1988 and, under subsequent legislation, all meat and milk from cattle suspected of having the disease is destroyed and prevented from entering the food chain.

BSE is a food-borne disease caused by bacteria that are highly resistant to heat. Whereas there is concern that humans could contact BSE through handling or eating meat products from infected cows, there is no evidence at present that BSE can be transmitted to humans. Most expert opinion consider the risk to humans negligible.

The Bovine Offal (Prohibition) Regulations 1989 prohibits certain offals (from all cattle) in food products intended for human consumption. These are: brain, spinal cord, spleen, thymus, tonsil and intestines. It is considered unlikely that young animals pose a risk from BSE to humans and these offals can be used in meat products if they come from calves under six months of age.

Government figures published in June 1992 showed that the total confirmed cases of BSE in the UK were more than 55,000. There were on average 631 new cases each week up to June 1992, compared to 437 each week in 1991. This is an increase of 45%. The total number of confirmed cases since the disease was first recorded in 1986 amounted to 55,300 to the end of April 1992.

Tapeworms and Cysteriosis

Tapeworms are a group of intestinal parasitic worms. Each consists of a tiny head and a neck region which produces segments. These enlarge as the worm grows and break off as the worm matures. The worm can grow up to 30 foot long, being attached to the wall of the bowel by hooks or suckers on its head; the mature segments are passed in the faeces.

The common tapeworm of man is caught from undercooked pork, beef or fish. The adult tapeworm from beef or pork causes no symptoms, except for the disgust the victim feels when passing the segments. Occasionally the fish tape worm causes anaemia because it competes with the victim for a B vitamin needed for the formation of red blood cells. The life-cycle of tapeworms involves the formation of cystic larvae in the tissues of the animal host. The larvae of the fish and beef tapeworm never develop in man, but those of the pork tapeworm may do so giving rise to cysteriosis. If the brain is affected epilepsy or even death may occur. There are effective drugs to remove tapeworms but no known treatment for cysteriosis.

DO cook all meat products thoroughly to kill bacteria and any cysts present.
DO NOT cook chickens from frozen, defrost them completely.
DO cook the stuffing separately from the bird.
DO refrigerate on delivery (from April 1993 at 0°C).
DO wash hands before and after handling food.
DO NOT allow raw meat to come into contact with other foods.
DO prepare a suitable clean surface used for raw meats only.
DO wash and sterilize all knives and equipment immediately after use.
DO NOT part cook joints of meat one day and complete cooking them the next day.

Eggs

Eggs are a high-risk food, a food which is unusually high in protein and moisture will encourage the growth of bacteria. Raw egg is ideal for bacterial growth and the shell may be contaminated with bacteria which will be transferred to the hand. During 1988 and 1989 there was a great deal of media attention concerning salmonella food poisoning and raw eggs. This problem is of course nothing new. During World War II dried egg from the USA was used by housewives in Great Britain who would make up a mixture of dried egg and milk, leave it overnight and then cook it quickly in the morning for breakfast. Illness from food poisoning resulted. But there has been a real increase in the number of cases associated with salmonella-infected eggs. In the first three months of 1989 there were 1,500 (UK) reported cases of food poisoning caused by the salmonella strain enteriditis phage type-4 associated with eggs and probably ten times as many cases went unreported.

Eggs become infected in three ways. There may be bacteria on the shell which may get inside the egg when the shell is cracked or broken; the bacteria may be inside the hen and be implanted in the egg before it is laid; bacteria can be absorbed through the shell. The bacteria is easily killed by cooking. At 70°C nearly all the bacteria are killed in three to four minutes. Modern methods for certain caterers mean that pasteurized eggs should be used, e.g. cake decoraters using pasteurized egg whites for icing cakes.

An outbreak of salmonella food poisoning was confirmed in July 1992 and following an investigation by an EHO the source was traced to eggs bought from a market stall. Five people were taken ill, three victims were admitted to hospital. All were previously fit, healthy young men who trained at the same gym. The eggs were mixed into drinks and drunk raw. This practice is believed to be widespread and the local council has written to all gyms warning them of the risks involved with raw eggs.

DO wash hands before and after handling raw eggs.
DO discard any eggs with cracked shells.
DO store eggs in a refrigerator.
DO eat cooked eggs and their products as soon as possible after preparation or refrigerate. Use within two days.
DO buy from a reputable supplier and buy clean-looking eggs.
DO cook eggs until the yolk and the white is set, six minutes boiling. The yolk solidifes at a higher temperature than the white at 70°C.
DO make egg sauces (hollandaise or bearnaise) in small batches, or to order so that they are not left in warm kitchens for a long time.
DO prepare any dishes which contain lightly cooked egg carefully and in small batches.
DO NOT use raw egg.

DO NOT use raw shell.
DO NOT serve eggs 'sunny side up'. Baste fried eggs in fat until the yolk is firm or turn the eggs over.
DO NOT store dishes with a meringue topping, eat them the same day or throw away.
DO NOT serve high-risk dishes to high-risk groups.

Milk
Milk is classed as a high-risk food but should not pose a problem so long as pasteurized or sterilized milk and correct storage conditions are used.

Ice-cream
The Milk Marketing Board (MME) has issued a Code of Practice on the hygienic production of ice-cream and related products. The Code is aimed at small- and medium-sized manufacturers and was drawn up because it is important for the ice-cream industry to be seen to be tightening up on hygiene. If you make ice-cream for someone else to consume you have to comply with regulations. If you sell to a third party the ice-cream must be pasteurized. If you are buying in, buy from a reputable supplier, never refreeze. Commercial ice-creams must be stored at –20°C immediately on delivery. If the product has been allowed to defrost it must be thrown away. Ice-cream scoops must be kept in a sterilant between service, which should be changed regularly.

Fish
Freshly cooked fish is rarely implicated in food poisoning outbreaks but they are classed as high-risk foods since fish decomposes more rapidly than meat and other perishable foods. Bacteria are not usually present in the intestines of cold-blooded animals, but care must be taken during preparation and storage as they are high in protein and moisture and will encourage the growth of food poisoning bacteria.

DO wash all fish before filleting and before preparation.
DO remove the slime present on fresh fish and wash out the gills to remove mud and slime.

DO clean down work surfaces after gutting and clear away the offal.
DO place on clean trays and refrigerate at 1°-2°C until needed.
DO store whole fish (before preparation) at 0°C with wet ice to keep it both moist and cold.

Game

Although meat and therefore high-risk, game has been the subject of a different, traditional method of storing and cooking. Game, such as pheasant, grouse and hare, which is hung for some time before cooking, must be thoroughly cooked before serving because of the increased risk of contamination associated with these methods. It will probably arrive at your premises complete with feathers, fur and innards intact.

The presence of lead shot is unlikely to give rise to an offence under Section 14 Food Safety Act 1990 as it can reasonably be expected to be there.

DO ensure a separate area is kept specifically for plucking, skinning and eviscerating. The fur may be infested with fleas and other insects and the feet may be dirty.
DO take care when handling any meat, poultry or game not to scratch the hands. This can cause infections, e.g. tetanus.

Fruit and Vegetables

Although fruit and vegetables are low-risk foods and do not provide the ideal conditions for bacterial growth, they can be affected by toxic sprays, and by pesticides used to disinfest crops. Salads that are eaten raw should be cleaned thoroughly before use. Some plants contain natural substances which are poisonous to humans, and there were 40,000 cases of plant poisoning in 1991. Some plants that are poisonous are: hemlock, deadly nightshade, laburnum leaves and seeds, foxglove and, the most common cause of vegetable food poisoning, toadstools mistaken for mushrooms or indeed some varieties of mushrooms.

Apples going brown can lead to increasing amounts of a mould called peniculiium expansum, which produces patulin. There is evidence that high levels of patulin can cause cancer and damage the immune, nervous and gastro-intestinal systems. It is worth emphasizing that individuals would have to consume huge amounts over a long period of time.

There are certain points to consider when handling, storing and preparing fruit and vegetables.

DO select fruit and vegetables from a reputable supplier.
DO store correctly in clean, airy conditions.
DO inspect daily and throw away any rotting or mouldy items.
DO wash all fruit and vegetable under cold running water to remove all soil. Soil will contain Cl. perfringens spores. This includes salad vegetables which, even if they look clean and may be shrink wrapped in plastic, must still be washed. This will also remove any pesticide residue.
DO wash before they arrive in the cooking area.
DO store under refrigeration temperatures. This will give them a longer practicable storage life.
DO ensure adequate storage ventilation during storage. This prevents condensation and mould growing. Apples and pears require perforated packaging to provide ventilation and avoid fermentation.
DO avoid buying all vegetables with excessive soil adhering. This could mean possible contamination with bacillus cereus and cl. botulinum.
DO NOT use potatoes with frost damage or those that have been exposed to light and have gone green. This may produce solanine poisoning.
DO wash all lettuce and cabbage thoroughly to remove soil and echinococcus cysts (caused by the tapeworm that dogs carry) and store all vegetables at least eighteen inches off the ground.
DO NOT buy fruit and nuts that are decomposing since this could be due to parasites.

LOW-RISK FOODS

Low-risk foods are foods that usually do not support bacterial growth, i.e. those with a pH value of less than 4.5. Foods with a high concentration of sugar, salt, acid, fat or dry foods do not provide moisture or proteins and are therefore not ideal for the growth of food poisoning bacteria (e.g. jams, syrups, honey, salted meat and anchovies). The sugar/salt concentration is too high for bacterial growth because the sugar and salt dissolve in the water to give a concentrated solution without sufficient moisture.

Fatty Foods

Food poisoning bacteria will not multiply in the presence of high concentrations of fat.

Acid Foods

Food poisoning bacteria will not grow in foods that are high in acid, e.g. pickles, citrus food.

Dry Foods

Rice and dried milk products, for example, may contain food poisoning bacteria, but as moisture is one of the conditions of bacterial growth the bacteria will not be growing and multiplying. When water is added to the food for mixing or cooking then treat the food as high risk and follow the rules of keeping food outside the 'danger zone'. Dried foods in packets should be put into containers to prevent insects and other pests gaining entry into the food. Place in clean plastic or glass containers with lids and store on shelving off the floor.

Canned foods during manufacture are canned and sterilized under strict control and will not normally support bacterial growth. However if the can is damaged, for example if the can is punctured or bulging or has a faulty seam, the manufacturer should be notified and the contents returned or thrown away.

PRESERVATION OF FOODS

Most of the methods devised for keeping the food safe (preservation) are concerned with controlling the bacteria and moulds in food.

Preservatives

As well as heat and cold, chemicals such as salt, nitrate, acid and other preserving substances are used. Permitted preservatives include:

Ascorbic used in flour, confectionery, cheese, maripan etc.
Benzoic acids used in soft fruit pulps, drinking coffee etc.
Sulphur dioxide added to sausages, mince meat, dehydrated vegetables, fruits, drinks etc.

PRESERVATION METHODS IN COMMON USE:
Accelerated freeze drying.
Antibiotics.
Bacterial preserving.
Deep freezing.
Dehydration, e.g. milk powder.
Heat treatment.
Immersion in brine or salt solution, e.g. bacon.
Smoking and curing.

There are problems associated with these methods of preserving. for example, contamination of the brine solution; under-processing of canned foods; the use of contaminated water for cooking purposes; freezing of already contaminated foods, e.g. salmonella in chickens; inadequate thawing before cooking; the fact that since dehydration may not destroy all micro-organisms, the addition of water may stimulate bacterial growth; the possible increase of antibiotic resistant strains of bacteria; and the risk of allergy. Food storage must be correct.

Natural Drying
This reduces the moisture level so that the bacteria cannot grow and the chemical processes are almost stopped. Food dried this way (e.g. prunes, dates, figs, currants) cannot normally be reconstituted. The product is still subject to insect pests if stored for a long time.

Freeze Drying
Freezing the food and then drying it by cold air blasts is a very effective method. The food can be reconstituted and is suitable for the mass freezing of vegetables.

Drying by Artificial Heat
This alters the food since it is cooked as well as dried. Some liquid foods, e.g. milk, are dried by spraying in hot air or a thin film over a heated roller. In all cases the food has to have less than 5% moisture to be effective; powders are usually less than 1%.

Canning
Food after canning should be sterile and will keep indefinitely. The stages in canning are:

1 The food is trimmed and prepared by blanching; this reduces the air in food and kills the enzymes on the surface.
2 The food is filled into cans and the air left above the food is removed by vacuum or by replacing it with steam. This is the usual method.
3 The lid is put on and then sealed.
4 The whole can is cooked for up to 45 minutes in a pressure cooker to kill all the bacteria. The object is to kill any clostridium botulinum which may be present. Cooking times vary from 330 minutes at 100°C to four minutes in a pressure cooker.

Bacterial Preserving
Natural preserving uses the bacteria, e.g. yoghurt, sauerkraut. In this method special bacteria are added to start fermentation. They also produce acid and eventually acid levels rise until the bacteria can no longer live. If controlled this occurs before the food is destroyed and the result is a preserved food which is different from the original, in the way that yoghurt is not the same as milk.

Vacuum Packing
All the air is drawn out of the container, usually plastic bags, and then sealed. This food has only a short life as chemical changes can still take place.

Inert Gas (usually Nitrogen)
The air is replaced by nitrogen and these products last a little longer than those that are vacuum-packed.

Irradiation

Irradiation sterilizes the food, but it still needs packing in sealed containers to prevent bacteria recontaminating.

Strict controls are placed on additives in food. Any excess or use of additives not permitted will automatically render the food 'unfit' and it can be seized and destroyed. Examples of preservative additions include:

Sulphur dioxide – in sausages.
Benzoic acid – in beer.
Proprinoic acid – in bread.
Antioxidents – prevents rancidity in edible fats.
Emulsifiers – for the even distribution of fats, cheese etc.
Solvents – used to carry ingredients, e.g. colours, preservative etc. Normally alcohols or glycerols, the types and purity are controlled and tested regularly.

Most metallic compounds are poisonous, but are naturally present in food as the plants pick up metals from the soil. Animals and fish feed from the plants and there are strict maximum limits on the amounts of lead, copper, metal, tin, arsenic, zinc and antimony that may be present.

Pesticides and insecticides. Both are used by farmers to prevent crops being destroyed by pests. Maximum limits are set and foods declared unfit if the levels are too high. Fruit and vegetables are usually affected and it can be dangerous if the food is eaten uncooked.

Pasteurization

In the nineteenth century Louis Pasteur developed methods of growing bacteria in a laboratory, and he proved beyond doubt that bacteria was the cause of disease. One aspect of his work, which is important in the study of food hygiene, is that he was able to show clearly that if a food product was sterilized by thorough cooking, living bacteria would not appear in the food unless they came from outside, either from the air, hands or other infected material.

The aim of pasteurization is to destroy the pathogens, without necessarily killing all the bacteria. At the same time, by reducing the temperature and time for which food has to be heated, changes in flavour and appearance are kept to a minimum. This applies to milk, ice-cream, liquid eggs and certain cooked meats (which for commercial reasons it may be impossible or impracticable to sterilize). Most modern dairies pasteurize milk using the continuous flow system, which utilizes the High Temperature Short Time (HTST) method. The supply of milk is pumped through a filter into heat exchanges where it is warmed to a temperature of 71.3°C and retained at that level for several seconds. They are then required to reduce the temperature to 10°C at the other end of the machine. It is required by law that indicating and recording thermometers be provided so that inspectors can see that each batch is being correctly treated. A flow diversion valve also returns to the start any milk which is not at the correct temperature.

Ice-cream mix must either be pasteurized or sterilized. A number of different time and temperature combinations are used.

Liquid eggs used for baking or for the manufacture of dried egg must be pasteurized, usually at a temperature of 64.9°C for 2½ minutes.

Pasteurization is carried out to certain large cans of meat, where sterilization would use too much heat and cause damage to the meat. The can is usually labeled 'to be kept under refrigeration'.

Sterilization is aimed at killing all the bacteria. This applies mainly to canned foods, milk and certain ice-cream mixes. The time and temperature combination for the sterilization of canned foods depends upon the nature of the food itself, the type of the pack and size of the pack. The principle of the process is to ensure that the entire mass of the meat reaches a temperature above boiling point. The main bacteria that canners are concerned with is clostridium botulinum. For this reason most canned foods are heated at temperatures around 115.5°C for a period of several minutes, but it is not possible to generalize.

As far as milk is concerned there are again variations of time and temperature. In the batch method, the milk is heated to approximately 115.5°C for 20 minutes in bottles that have already been sealed. The milk will keep for long periods until opened, but the milk sugars are caramelized by the heat and it has a characteristic flavour. To obviate the unpleasant flavour Ultra Heat Treatment (UHT) was devised. This is a continuous flow process where the milk is heated to 132°C for one second before sterile bottling. This milk is often called 'Long Life Milk'. Ice-cream is sterilized in a similar matter at a temperature of approximately 149°C for two seconds after which it is dried and packed.

Irradiation of Food

Irradiation of food has been investigated for the last thirty years. In the UK irradiated food was banned for twenty-four years and was only given Government clearance from 1 January 1991, subject to further legislation. Since October 1991, thirty-seven countries have had clearances to irradiate a range of food products intended for human consumption. The International Atomic Energy Agency say 'as of May 1991 there have been fifty-one food irradiation plants built and fifteen planned or awaiting completion throughout the world.' In the UK there is only one company, Isotron of Swindon, Wiltshire, that has been given a licence to irradiate and sell fourteen varieties of herbs and spices (June 1991) to the public. There are some irradiation plants in the UK for the non-food industry, e.g. for the manufacture of surgical instruments.

Irradiation differs totally from radioactive contamination and is intended to kill micro-organisms, particularly pathogenic micro-organisms. It is comparable to pasteurization and destroys spoilage organisms.

The product to be irradiated is given doses of ionizing radiation using radioactive substances such as cobalt-60 and caesium-137. These give out gamma rays. The doses are measured in grays (after the British radiobiologist, L.H. Gray who died in 1965).

1 gray = 1 joule per kg
1 kg = 1,000 grays.

Typical doses for food:

Up to one kilogray: Kills parasites in raw meat, insects, and slows sprouting in potatoes.
Up to ten kilograys: Kills bacteria (salmonella and campylobacter) in raw poultry and shellfish.

Over ten kilograys reduces bacterial count of herbs and spices.
Ten–twelve grays will kill a person within a few days, but some bacteria and viruses may survive 200,000 grays.

Gamma rays are used for irradiating foods, since they have more penetrating power than alpha and beta particles and can pass easily through food packaging. The UK Advisory Committee on Irradiation and Novel Foods has said: 'It is satisfied that irradiation poses no safety problems, provided doses given to foods do not exceed ten kilograys (10,000 grays) as at the energy levels proposed for food irradiation the amount of radioactivity is so small and dies away rapidly.' After food has been irradiated, enzymes are damaged and can no longer speed up chemical reactions, and DNA can no longer control the cells. The vitamin loss and reduction of nutritive value is only comparable to established methods of processing e.g. heat processing. It also produces some chemical changes in food, slightly affecting the carbohydrate, fats and protein molecules. Irradiating foods will destroy some micro-organisms leaving the food unaltered and this has been identified as an area of malpractice. In 1986 a company in the UK was prosecuted for exporting prawns to Holland for irradiating. The prawns had a higher than normal micro-biological load. The irradiated prawns were then re-imported with a corresponding low level of micro-organisms and treated as fresh. This process would not have destroyed any toxins that some bacteria can produce.

In other countries irradiation has replaced the use of chemicals in commercial operations. In Italy, Japan and Hungary, low level irradiation has been used for the inhibition of sprouting in potatoes. Ten countries are now using irradiation to treat herbs and spices to reduce bacterial levels. In the USA irradiation is used for the control of insects in grain and for some fruit crops. Holland is the pioneer in using irradiation on chickens, then freezing them. South Africa uses irradiation for treating fruit successfully, e.g. preventing mould in strawberries. Tropical fruits respond well. Ripening is retarded in some fruits and accelerated in others. White fish can be irradiated, but fatty foods (such as oily fish) may become rancid.

In 1979 the Hungarian Academy of Sciences carried out a study of food irradiation. They classified the results into three groups and found that 7,191 studies showed neutral effects, 185 had effects that were clearly beneficial and 1,414 showed adverse effects (vitamins destroyed or an altered taste).

Recent surveys carried out by the Food Commission's Food Irradiation Campaign found out that 84% of customers questioned would not buy irradiated food and 70% of large food manufacturers in the UK have said they would not use food irradiation for processing their products.

The EC have proposed new laws to provide free trade in irradiated foods after 1992 but there is opposition. There remains a great deal of uncertainty and disagreement on the subject of irradiating foods.

DANGER ZONE

Bacteria that produce food poisoning grow most rapidly at a temperature of around 37°C, body temperature, but as long as one of the conditions for growth, warmth, is present they will multiply in a vast range of temperatures. The temperatures that are ideal for bacterial growth are 5°C–63°C. For this reason the range of temperatures is called the 'danger zone'. Even a small number of bacteria will grow rapidly at these temperatures and soon become present in sufficient numbers to cause food poisoning. Temperatures outside the 'danger zone' are less suitable for the bacteria. Most bacteria are killed at 75°C while being cooked for 10–30 minutes. It is important to maintain this temperature in the centre of the food. However, some bacteria and their toxins need higher temperatures for a longer period of time before they are destroyed. In cold conditions, below 5°C, bacterial growth is slowed and virtually ceases. Some will die but the majority survive and grow again at 'danger zone' temperatures. Frozen foods contain food poisoning bacteria but the conditions are not right for the bacteria to grow.

Food that is being defrosted should be stored in a refrigerator, NOT at 'danger zone' temperatures.

DO ensure that cooked foods which are not required immediately are either cooled quickly and then refrigerated or kept hot at above 63°C.
DO NOT store food at 'danger zone' temperatures.

It is very often carelessness that allows bacteria the time they need. Food left in the 'danger zone' allows the bacteria to double their numbers every ten to twenty minutes. After twenty-four hours it is possible for one bacteria to increase in number to 7,000 million.

DO NOT allow bacteria the time to multiply.

TEMPERATURE CONTROL

Correct temperature control is vital to control the growth of bacteria. A report in 1986 showed that the majority of food poisoning cases were caused by careless temperature control.

The Food Hygiene (Amendment) Regulations 1990 have been introduced to specify chilled and hot temperature controls for certain foods. They identify foods which will support rapid multiplication of pathogenic bacteria present, if not adequately controlled by temperature. The regulations apply to the temperature of the foods, but in practice air temperature measurements will often be the means for monitoring the temperature of chilled foods once a relationship has been established between air and food temperatures. The regulations state:

Chilled foods are to be kept at below 8°C.

Hot foods are to be kept at above 63°C.

Food that is kept at or below 8°C may rise in temperature by not more than 2°C for not more than two hours.

Food Storage Temperatures
General purpose refrigerator 4°C.
Dairy refrigerator 4°C.
Raw meat refrigerator 0°C.
Raw fish refrigerator –1°C.
Ice-cream conservator –21°C.
Deep freeze: Frozen meat –21° to –18°C, frozen vegetables –15°C.

The effect of temperature on the growth of bacteria

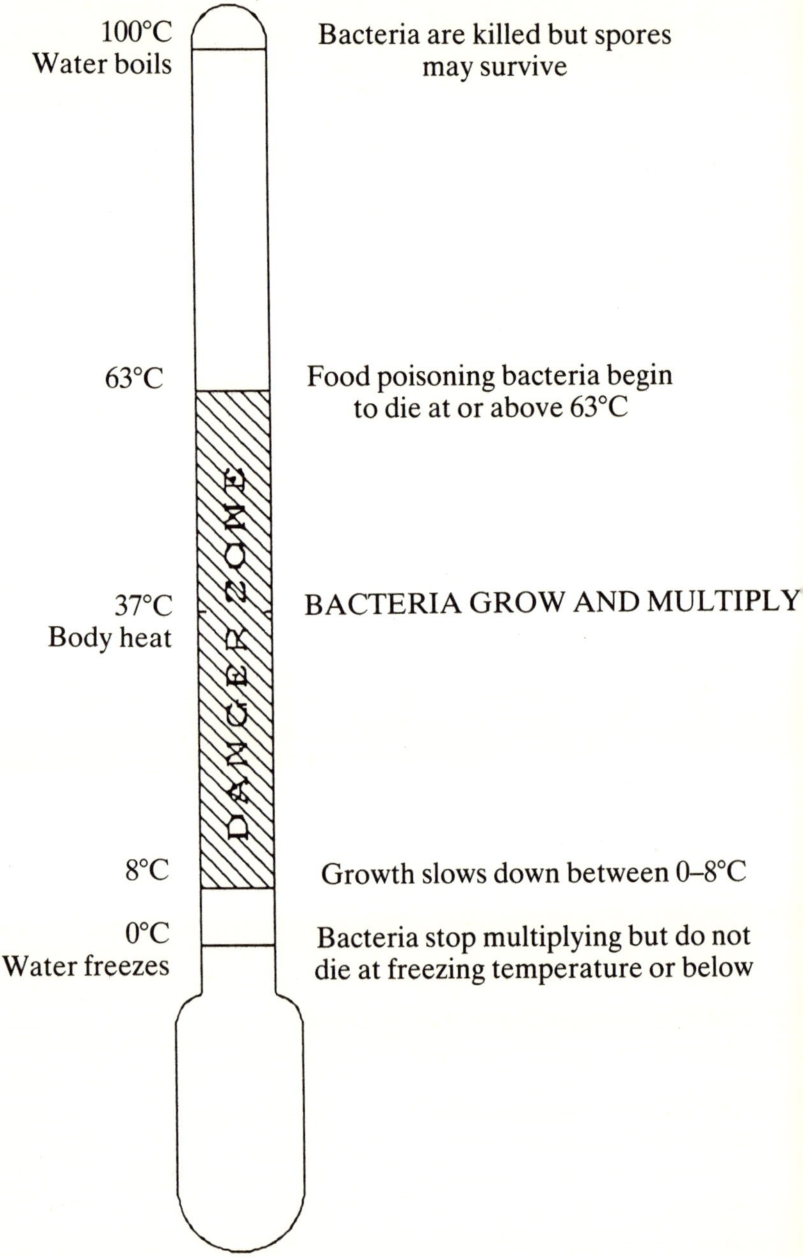
100°C
Water boils
Bacteria are killed but spores may survive
63°C
Food poisoning bacteria begin to die at or above 63°C
DANGER ZONE
37°C
Body heat
BACTERIA GROW AND MULTIPLY
8°C
Growth slows down between 0–8°C
0°C
Water freezes
Bacteria stop multiplying but do not die at freezing temperature or below

Correct use of refrigerator:

DO NOT overload. Cold air must be allowed to circulate.

DO store food below loading lines in display or chilled cabinets.

DO, where possible, use separate refrigerators for raw and cooked foods.

DO store raw foods below cooked foods.

DO defrost regularly.

DO check door seals or gaskets are in good repair.

DO secure an adhesive notice to each unit indicating what the unit is used for and the maximum operating temperatures (e.g. no. 1 4°C dairy). Place it where it can be easily seen.

DO install a permanent thermometer, accurate within 1°C, inside each unit.

DO check temperatures of each unit three times a day.

DO record the readings and keep the records.

Ambient Temperature

Ambient temperature is room temperature. Once cooked food and liquids can be cooled at room temperature, kept covered, then refrigerated, but there is a risk of further contamination. Open food should be discouraged. Food for sale must be kept covered or protected from risk of contamination. Protecting food in this way cuts down the risk of contamination from insects, dust and dirt, and from bacteria being coughed or sneezed on to it.

DO cover all food including food being stored and refrigerated.

DO ensure food on display is protected.

DO NOT leave food at room temperature for longer than 1½ hours.

DO keep covered during cooling time.

DO refrigerate after cooling until required.

DO NOT allow the general public to touch the food; protect food with a 'sneeze guard'.

COOKING

Food which is cooked fresh and eaten whilst hot should not

be the cause of food poisoning. Cooking will kill most bacteria that are present on the food in its raw state. If the bacteria are spore-forming and produce toxins, the spores will remain inactive after cooking if the food is kept at 63°C or refrigerated. Temperature control during the cooking process is vital.

If food is overcooked, the food will become spoiled or even burnt. An unskilled or inexperienced chef or cook will not produce good food, and may also risk poisoning the customers with contaminated food. They should be aware of the problems of both undercooking and overcooking food.

There are three frequent reasons why food is inadequately cooked:

Thawing Frozen Poultry and Joints of Meat

Any ice left inside the meat will slow down the cooking process. All the heat energy will go into melting the ice, not cooking the meat. The inside cavity of a frozen or partially defrosted chicken will spend some part of the cooking process in 'danger zone' temperatures. All poultry is regarded as hazardous because it is contaminated with salmonella. NEVER undercook poultry. The temperature inside the cavity should reach 75°C. Check the meat is cooked by inserting a skewer or a knife into the joint between the leg and the body, if the juices run clear with no blood in them the meat is cooked.

Cooking Too Large a Joint of Meat

The heat will penetrate too slowly into a large joint of meat, so limit the size to 3 kg maximum and use a probe thermometer to ensure a minimum centre temperature of 75°C.

Time and Temperature

The food has to spend a certain period of time at a temperature above 75°C to cook thoroughly. There are several reasons for the food not achieving this temperature: the person cooking the food is in a hurry and may lack understanding or have planned badly; the cooking technique is wrong for the type of food being cooked; customer preference; the failure of equipment.

Most types of modern equipment will ensure that the food is cooked thoroughly, e.g. forced air convection cookers, steam ovens, Bratt pans, pressure cookers and deep fat fryers. However other cooking equipment can pose some risks:

Conventional ovens use convection: heat rises and naturally circulates. The temperature across a shelf will be constant but the base shelf could be 30°C cooler than the top shelf. Temperature varies and an old or poorly maintained oven may not be working properly. Check the actual oven temperature. A fan-assisted oven with re-circulating air will help to maintain an even temperature.

Slow cookers are acceptable but the temperature should be checked to see if it eventually maintains a minimum 63°C throughout the food. When cooked, serve the food immediately. Leftover food should be discarded as cooking food at low temperatures for a long time might compromise the safety of the food you are cooking.

DO use a commercial slow cooker.
DO follow the manufacturer's instructions.
DO NOT overfill and make sure the recommended minimum cooking time is completed.
DO probe test the final temperature of the food. Slow cookers are designed to obtain an eventual minimum temperature of 63°C throughout the food. Anything lower would not be safe.
DO boil red kidney beans for fifteen minutes before adding to the slow cooking process.

Microwave ovens and under cooking. Dangers relate to the use of unsuitable containers, dense food, low wattage ovens and uneven cooking. Because foods do not brown, visual checks are not adequate.

During the cooking of large pans of liquids such as stocks, gravy, soups or stews, it is vital to maintain and ensure an even distribution of heat. This cooking method drives out air so that anaerobic bacteria present get the conditions they need to grow and multiply. Even though the surface liquid is boiling there may be cold spots in the liquid. It is vital to ensure there are no cold spots because spore-forming bacteria can reproduce at lower temperatures.

DO cook smaller batches. Split into two pans if necessary.
DO NOT cook more than twenty-five litres in bulk.
DO use wide low pans with a heat source equal to the width of the pan.
DO keep the lids on when the product is cooking.
DO stir the product frequently – at least every ten minutes.
DO ensure that the spoon used for stirring is not placed on a soiled surface. Put it across the pan, or on a clean plate at the side of the pan. Make sure the spoon is not in contact with the heat source.

Stock-pot

The stock-pot in a kitchen traditionally stays on the cooker throughout the day, and various items are added to the stock from time to time. Stock that has been boiling for several hours will not be the cause of food poisoning if it is served or used hot. If it has been kept warm and then reheated it is likely to cause problems. Decide whether to continue with the practice of keeping a stock-pot or use a commercially produced dry stock product. If you decide to continue with the stock-pot then:

DO ensure all contents are discarded daily and the pot thoroughly washed.
DO NOT add uncooked meats and DO NOT add unwashed vegetables.

Heated Display Units

A bain-marie (water-bath) is a heated well filled with water. The water must be heated to a temperature of at least 63°C and be capable of holding this temperature. For all hot display units:

DO NOT use units to heat up foods. The food must be hot before placing in the hot display.
DO clean units out every day.
DO throw away any food left in the containers at the end of the day and wash the container thoroughly.

Eighteen people were taken ill with a Christmas outbreak of salmonella food poisoning. They were amongst a group of sixty people who attended a Christmas function in a restaurant. The cooking procedures were described as 'ludicrous' by the Chief Environmental Health Officer. A 35 lb turkey used for the event had been cooked for only 3½ hours (as opposed to 12 hours at 20 mins per lb and 20 mins over). It had then been left for 24 hours at room temperature and warmed through before serving. 'Luckily no one had to be taken to hospital, as there were no people in the high-risk/old age group, who are most at risk from dying if they suffer from food poisoning.'

DO ensure staff are trained in cooking methods.
DO insist on frozen joints and poultry being properly thawed.
DO check sizes of joints for cooking.
DO ensure food is cooked for long enough at a high enough temperature.

Cook-Chill
This is a method of food preparation that is used widely in hospitals, for school meals and inflight meals and is now also widely available in all major supermarket outlets in the UK. The food is prepared in a Central Production Unit (CPU) where the food is cooked and portioned into individual containers. These containers are then date-coded and labelled with the reheating instructions and the contents. The product undergoes an initial heating process and is then held at 0°C–4°C. It must be held at this temperature before, during and after distribution and reheated to a temperature of at least 70°C within two hours of its arrival at the point of consumption. The refrigeration stage should not exceed five days.

There have been a number of worrying contraventions of the current Department of Health (DHSS) Guidelines 1981. The recently reported isolation of listeria in cook-chill products is worrying at least one manufacturer who supplies cook-chill products with a shelf life of seven days to major supermarkets. The packages state 'eat within two days of purchase'. Assuming that such a product may not appear on a shelf until three days after manufacture the product can be up to twelve days old before being eaten. Many thermometers in refrigerated display units in supermarkets consistently show temperatures exceeding 5°C, which according to the guidelines would require the destruction of the chilled products being held.

Hazard analysis with microbiological sampling of all cook-chill products should be undertaken by all commercial cook-chill producers.

Listeria has been found in commercial cook-chill products but there has been no comparative study of cook-chill meals from a hospital CPU. Department of Health (DOH) guidelines recommend the sampling for salmonella and staphylococus aureus, but no recommendation is made for listeria. Of all groups of high risk people, hospital patients are the ones who would be most at risk from listeriosis. With reference to cook-chill products the following recommendations have been put forward:

Listeriosis should be made a notifiable disease.

Cook-chill products should not be kept at refrigerated conditions for more than three days.

Retail outlets should comply with DOH guidelines and remove from sale and destroy products whose temperatures are found to be held above 4°C by probe testing the product, not by measuring the temperature of the ventilating area.

The DOH guidelines should be amended to include listeria in the microbiological monitoring of cook-chill products.

The reheating of cook-chill products should be shown to destroy all listeria that may be present.

The introduction of cook-chill catering should be suspended until the safety of the system can be shown.

Until the above recommendations can be implemented any refrigerated foods found to contain listeria in twenty-five grammes should be declared unfit for human consumption.

DO NOT forget that listeria comes from dirty working conditions. In most cases the food handler with poor hygiene standards is reponsible for introducting the listeria into otherwise clean food.

Cooling or Chilling

Cooling or chilling is designed to take the heat out of food by reducing the temperature. This is not the same as refrigerating for holding or storage purposes, but it is designed to hold food at its final temperature. Heat removal (e.g. blast chillers or blast freezers) operates at air velocity, which is too high for the storage of foods, as the food will dry out.

Refrigerators or chill rooms only cope with small heat changes, such as opening the door.

Sous Vide

The last few years has seen the introduction of *sous vide* into catering operations, whereby the food product is put into vacuum-packed bags and then sold to the customer to take away. The food is subsequently reheated before being consumed.

The food is put into the bag, a cryovac pouch which is either a shrink pouch which clings to the food or is non shrink for food items such as fish. A vacuum-packaging machine draws out 99% of the air and seals the pack. The pack is then put into a combination steam oven which allows cooking at temperatures below 100°C. A special steam controller ensures each type of food is cooked at the right temperature for the right length of time. After cooking the pack must be cooled rapidly. Smaller operations may use iced-water chillers but mass producers must use a blast chiller. After chilling the packs are labelled with the name of the product, the production date, the expiry date, the storage temperature, and reheating instructions. The pack must be stored at 0°C–2°C.

For reheating, the pack must be steamed and heated until it reaches 70°C, and then cut open and served.

The whole process is the development of the classic French method of cooking *en paillote* (steam cooking in an envelope). The method conserves the texture, flavour and colour of the food, and when stored correctly the product stays fresh and safe for up to six days.

Legislation is proposed for premises to be 'registered' to provide this service since the temperature control of food handled this way is very important. Extracting air from the pack provides anaerobic conditions for some bacteria, including clostridium botulinum, allowing them to multiply if food standards are poor.

DO prepare the recipes separately to cut down the risk of cross contamination.
DO use good quality fresh foods.
DO ensure top quality machinery for vacuum packing.
DO ensure strict temperature controls on cooking and storage.
DO label the pack carefully with reheating times and temperatures.
DO NOT save reheated foods. Throw them away.

Reheating

Reheating foods is a common practice in many catering establishments. If you apply the letter of the law the advice is to try and avoid reheating foods, but establishments will often batch cook, then portion down to enable the product to be reheated at a later date. To comply with current legislation follow these points.

Ensure the food to be stored in a refrigerator is thoroughly cooked.

Portion down and cool quickly. Keep the food covered during the cooling down period.

Refrigerate at 0–4°C. Five days is the maximum for the food to be stored, including the day it was cooked and the day it was reheated.

All foods to be reheated should be heated until piping hot and have an internal temperature of 70–75°C.

Most caterers now use microwave ovens to reheat cooked portions of food. If the product is larger than a single portion, e.g. a pan of chilli con carne, first reheat on a low heat (to prevent sticking or burning), raise the heat until boiling and stir frequently to ensure the heat is distributed throughout the food.

Defrosting

When thawing frozen foods, any bacteria present in the food in its frozen state will begin to multiply at temperatures above 0°C. If the food was safely cooked and cooled before freezing, the numbers of bacteria present will not be large; but if the food has been poorly handled before freezing, there is a greater risk of large numbers of bacteria and, during defrosting, the numbers could become sufficient to cause food poisoning. Various factors affect defrosting time.

Defrosting is quicker if the product is small, chicken portions will defrost quicker than a whole bird. Vegetables will defrost quickly and should be cooked from frozen.

Tightly packed and vacuum-packed foods will defrost as quickly as wrapped foods, but unwrapped foods lead to drying and discolouration of the product. Loose packing will trap air and increase thawing times.

Moving air under water will defrost frozen foods faster than air and water that cannot circulate.

Refrigeration temperatures are ideal for defrosting. It is a slower and safer method of defrosting as the food will not spend any time in the 'danger zone'. When defrosting food in the refrigerator, separate items that are frozen together as soon as they start to defrost to speed up the defrosting time. A fan-assisted refrigerator will also speed up defrosting time.

Most commercial microwave ovens have a defrost setting but food should not be entirely defrosted on this setting since the microwave energy will start to cook the food's outer layer before the centre is defrosted.

DELIVERY AND DELIVERY VEHICLES

All deliveries should be checked on arrival at your premises. All dried goods and canned goods should be visibly checked for damage to boxes, cartons and containers. If the containers are damaged they may have been dropped, damaging the cans inside or even the contents of the cans. Visible damage may have occured some time ago, allowing pests to gain access to the food product.

If the delivery contains frozen products, it is advisable to keep a delivery record. The information recorded will enable accurate checks on the suitability of the supplier. The packaging should be visibly checked together with the temperature of the frozen food at the time of delivery. If the temperature is unacceptable then the product should be rejected. DO NOT refreeze.

Delivery vehicles are covered by the Food Hygiene (Markets, Stalls and Delivery Vehicle) Regulations 1966 and the temperature control of these vehicles has been amended by the Food Hygiene (Amendment) Regulations 1990. These changes allow foods to be delivered at a higher temperature than their specified storage temperature under certain conditions depending on the size of the vehicle and the journey distance:

Over 7.5 tonnes and carrying food outside their locality, must deliver all relevant foods at no more than 8°C (from 1 April 1991). From 1 April 1993 not more than 5°C.

Under 7.5 tonnes and local deliveries should deliver relevant food at 8°C from 1 April 1992. Small vehicles can continue at this temperature even after 1 April 1993. If foods are delivered above the storage temperature, store without further delay and fill in the record sheet.

Any vehicle used for transporting food for the purposes of a food business is subject to these requirements. Using a car to go to the cash and carry to collect goods makes that car a delivery vehicle. If collecting relevant foods, it becomes subject to temperature control requirements, so carry a cold box and ice packs to enable temperature controls to be kept on short journeys.

DO use delivery monitoring records to prove 'due diligence'.

DO NOT accept goods that are damaged or frozen goods that are defrosting.

DO buy frozen foods from a reputable supplier and check all incoming frozen deliveries for quality and temperature.

DO defrost bulk items of meat and poultry before cooking and serving.

DO defrost food items in containers that will contain any defrosting liquids and keep frozen foods away from cooked foods. Treat as raw meat. The liquid will contain bacteria. Defrost high-risk foods in the bottom of the refrigerator so that no liquids can drip onto clean food.

DO check food is thoroughly defrosted. The flesh should be pliable, there should be no ice crystals in the body cavity of poultry. Remove giblets as soon as possible, probe test for temperature. All parts of the food should not be lower than –1°C before cooking.

DO NOT defrost at room temperature. This method carries a higher risk of dangerous levels of bacteria multiplying in sufficient numbers to cause food poisoning.

TAKE-AWAY RESTAURANTS

Sandwiches

If preparing fillings in advance they should be individually wrapped and kept refrigerated below 8°C. If they are not sold after twelve hours – throw them away. The relevant food fillings must be kept at 2–4°C, especially: cooked sliced meats, meat pâtés, egg mayonnaise, prawns, crab, tuna and salmon. If sandwiches are made to order, the work surfaces must only be used for making sandwiches.

DO keep fillings refrigerated until required.
DO clean and dry knives after each order.

Salads

DO keep salads refrigerated whilst on display.
DO protect salads from risk of contamination. Keep them covered or use a display unit with a sneeze guard.
DO throw away any prepared salads not used by the end of the working day.

Fried Chicken Take-away

When frozen chicken portions are cooked by deep frying the internal temperature must reach 70–85°C, or there is a HIGH risk of food poisoning.

Spit Roasting Chicken

DO NOT leave chickens on the spit with the heat turned off.
DO keep uncooked chickens at 2–4°C until required for cooking.
DO defrost frozen chickens thoroughly.
DO store frozen chicken pieces at –20°C.
DO store chilled chicken pieces at 1–3°C and check expiry dates.
DO throw away any unused, unsold cooked chicken pieces at the end of the day.

Doner Kebabs

These defy all basic food hygiene procedures and need very careful handling. The recipe of lamb and spices is often a closely guarded secret and I know of at least one producer who uses a bath to mould the mixture together! It is a large joint (often 45 kg) and hygiene advice is not to cook a joint bigger than 3 kg to ensure thorough cooking. As a minced meat product, bacteria is minced throughout the product. It is difficult to refrigerate and will often be returned to the freezer to enable it to keep its characteristic shape.

Staff need training to cut the meat into slices, as the heat on the spit will only ever cook the outside layer of the meat and the underneath layer will be raw.

The slices are often reheated.

The grill is often turned down or off to prevent the meat burning when the customer demand is low at slack times.

DO refrigerate the meat before moulding.
DO wash hands and equipment before and after mixing and moulding.
DO use/make smaller kebabs.
DO use a special knife, just for cutting doner kebab and DO NOT use for any other food preparation.
DO wash the knife thoroughly between slicing.
DO serve the meat at once and DO NOT keep it warm.
DO NOT turn the heat off during quiet times.
DO NOT cut thick layers of kebab meat.

Indian and Chinese Take-aways
The biggest problems occur with batch cooked rice. Traditionally rice is cooked in advance, not refrigerated, and quickly stir-fried or refreshed to order.

Pizza
The base of the dough is no real problem as it is cooked at a high temperature and, because it is thin, the dough quickly reaches 70–85°C.

Check that the wide range of fillings and toppings are kept refrigerated until needed.

STANDARDS OF FOODS

Many foods have standards because of the amount of ingredients used. Food that does not contain the correct amount is not regarded as unfit for human consumption, but it is an offence which carries a fine. Meat pies must contain 25% meat, sausage rolls 12½% meat, luncheon meat 80% meat, beefburgers 80% meat, sausages (50% for beef 65% for pork), soft drinks (juice and sugar are controlled), fishcakes 35% fish, meat/fish paste 7%, and margarine must have vitamin A and 760–940 international units vitamin D.

DATE-CODING

The Food Labelling Regulations 1984 (As Amended) requires all food products delivered to catering establishments and consumers to carry a date code, except for certain products such as fresh fruit and vegetables, bread etc. All supplied food products that are susceptible to bacterial spoilage, including products which need to be refrigerated, must have the words 'Use By' followed by a date and recommended storage conditions. The 'Use By' date can be expressed as a day and a month, or as a day, month and a year.

These date-coding regulations now apply (from 20 June 1992) to cheese that is intended to ripen in its wrapper, either completely or partially. Under Section 40 of the Food Labelling Regulations 1984 'it is an offence to sell any food after its use by date or to alter the date code from its original.'

Sell By Dates

It is now compulsory for most foods to be date-marked. The main exceptions are 'long-life' foods, fresh fruit and vegetables and bread. The date mark is based on the durability of the food, that is the period of time which the manufacturer expects the food to maintain its flavour and other qualities so long as it is properly stored. Usually the date mark has the words 'best before' followed by the day, month and year in that order.

Perishable foods (those intended to be eaten within six weeks of packing) have the words 'sell by' instead of 'best before'. The year may be omitted when the food will not remain at its best for longer than three months. Only the manufacturer can decide the date mark, bearing in mind the ingredients used, the type of processing and packaging and the likely speed of distribution. Although it is not an offence for a shopkeeper to sell a product after the sell by date, an offence has been committed if the food is unfit for human consumption, or if the shopkeeper removes or blacks out a sell by date.

MICROBIOLOGICAL STANDARDS

There is no legal requirement for caterers to test their products for microbiological safety, but the Food Safety Act 1990 does put the responsibility on the caterer for the food they sell, and checks should be made on the product. Before deciding whether to use microbiological testing, there are certain factors to consider:

The size of the business and the resources available. The larger the organization the greater the need for testing.

The kind of product produced. Is it high- or low-risk food?

Whether your supplier of goods for production is reliable, reputable and tests his products.

If it is decided to undertake microbiological testing, specialist help is available from food hygiene consultants and from suppliers already using quality control systems that include microbiological testing.

Microbiological standards provide a target to ensure that levels of micro-organisms are kept to a low level and good standards of food hygiene and safe food handling are maintained.

If the size of the business and the resources available make microbiological testing unwarranted, you can set your own standards and keep micro-organisms to a minimum by following these procedures:

DO keep raw foods separate from cooked foods. Use separate areas for storage and preparation of raw and cooked foods. Colour coding is helpful to enforce separation in all areas.

DO totally isolate raw chicken and cook it thoroughly.

DO ensure equipment and utensils are easy to clean and in good repair. Damaged and faulty equipment and utensils should be repaired or replaced.

DO ensure all food handlers maintain high standards of

personal hygiene, keep their hands clean and wear clean protective clothing, keep their hair covered and cover cuts and sores with waterproof dressings.

DO check refrigerators daily to ensure temperatures are being maintained.

DO remove waste food and dirt constantly from kitchen areas.

DO keep handling of food to a minimum.

DO check the building, inside and out, to exclude pest entry. Store food in pest-proof containers.

DO have separate washhand basins. Sinks should not be used for washing hands.

DO use disposable cloths for wiping down.

DO store all food, equipment and utensils off the floor.

DO organize time to ensure that the time food spends in the 'danger zone' is kept to a minimum.

FOOD PACKAGING

At present (1992) the legal requirement concerning food packaging in this country is 'that it should not spoil or make food unsafe to eat' (reg. 12).

New EC Legislation will be introduced to specify exactly what chemicals can be used in packaging and set limits on the amount of chemicals that can be transferred from packaging into food. Contaminants from plastics have been found in all sorts of food and constituents can also transfer from metal, paper and glass into food. Examples of hazardous food packaging are:

Lead

Contamination by lead used to be far more common than it is now, especially with canned foods. There is still a small proportion of imported cans that use a lead solder to seal cans, but this problem is small. With lead closures on wine bottles, studies have shown that lead can get into the wine as it is being poured, lead can corrode and leave deposits on the neck of the bottle. Use a damp cloth or paper towel to wipe the neck and rim of the bottle before pouring.

DO NOT put lead crystal in a microwave.

Tin

Once a tin is opened, if the contents of the can are not to be used at once, put the contents into another container. Once the can is opened, the air, and the food itself, will attack the can coating, making the food unsafe.

Printed Plastics

Few plastics are designed for food use, and some coloured plastics contain toxic metals like cadmium. Never use printed bags turned inside out for food use, chemicals from the ink can transfer to food. You must only use plastics intended for food or those which are labelled 'for food use'. Only use plastic containers labelled 'microwave safe' or those obviously intended for microwave cooking. Plastic containers that are re-usable such as margarine tubs and ice-cream containers should not be used in a microwave to reheat food. Although they may not melt, harmful chemicals may still transfer to the hot food.

Wax

Mineral hydrocarbons are substances ranging from oily liquids to waxy solids. COT, the Government's Committee on Toxicity, says the 'evidence suggest, possible toxicity'. Mineral hydrocarbons are used in chewing gum, the coatings on some dried fruit, the rind on cheese like Edam and the peel of some citrus fruits (if it is labelled unwaxed, it has not been treated with mineral hydrocarbons).

Cling Films

There are two types of plastics used for the manufacture of cling film: PVC or polythene (known as non-PVC) and VDC Copolymer (known as microwave or freezer wrap). There is no evidence of a health hazard from any cling film or microwave and freezer wrap, but the COT, who are the advisors on the safety of chemicals in foods, has advised that too little is known about some of the chemicals that transfer from this film into wrapped food. They recommend that until more is known about these chemicals and safety levels can be set, it is sensible to limit the amount of them that is used and ingested.

Tests done by the Ministry of Agriculture, Fisheries and

Food in 1986 showed that the constituents of cling film leaked into food when it was used for microwave cooking. They stressed that this posed no risk to health, but still advised that it should not come into contact with food during cooking in a microwave or conventional oven. Manufacturers developed low migration cling film, in which fewer constituents leaked out. In November 1990 the Government published further research showing that chemicals from all cling film leaked into wrapped food, especially fatty food, even when cold. MAFF added a recommendation that cling film should not be used to wrap high fat foods.

DO NOT use cling film for wrapping fatty foods, e.g. cheese, butter, cooked meats, raw meats, oily fish, pastries and croissants, biscuits or cakes with chocolate and cream fillings, and sandwiches with fatty fillings like mayonnaise.
DO use, instead, dishes covered with cling film so that the film does not touch the food, or sealable plastic, glass containers, plastic bags or foil.
DO NOT use cling film in microwave cooking where the film touches the food.
DO NOT use cling film in conventional cookers, ovens with infra-red or combination ovens.
DO NOT buy fatty foods pre-wrapped in clinging plastic film.

At present cling films do comply with an EC directive on plastics, which is due to come into force fully in 1993, and it is now possible to buy a non-PVC type cling film.

HAZARD ANALYSIS AND CRITICAL CONTROL POINTS (HACCP) AND RISK ASSESSMENT

HACCP is a system to prevent problems by using the operation of identifying and grading risks so that resources can be effectively targeted. The system was devised in 1973 by NASA, Pilsbury and the US Army as a ‘nil defects programme’. It would have been a nonsense to send astronauts into space with contaminated foods that would have given them food poisoning. The aim of the programme is to identify hazards which happen in food preparation and to devise methods of controlling bacterial growth to ensure food safety by analysing the hazards, identifying the risks and controlling and monitoring the system.

Risk Assessment
In food production, risk assessment programmes are based on the assessment of risks that premises may fail to meet food standards by the composition of food, labelling standards and methods of preparation.

DUSTBINS AND WASTE DISPOSAL

Food waste provides ideal conditions for the growth of bacteria and, unless waste is dealt with properly (by containing it in a waste unit), it will attract insects and rodents, so that clean food is at risk from contamination. Waste food and dirt should be removed throughout the working day and must not be allowed to accumulate.

Internal waste units inside the food area should be operated by a food pedal. All containers should be fitted with a close-fitting lid, and the lid must be used. There should be sufficient numbers of waste units for the size of the business.

There should be a special area set aside, outside, for bins containing refuse and awaiting collection. Again they should have tight-fitting lids, so that pests cannot gain access to the waste. You must arrange for the bins to be emptied frequently. They must be placed on a suitable hard standing with facilities for washing down and disinfecting the area.

From 1 April 1992 the new law on waste, the Duty of Care, means that all reasonable steps must be taken to look after any waste, and prevent illegal disposal by others. There is an unlimited fine if this law is broken.

The Duty of Care
If someone produces, imports, stores, treats, processes, transports, recycles or disposes of controlled waste, the Duty of Care applies to them. (Controlled waste is any household, commercial or industrial waste from a house, shop, factory, building site or any other business premises.) Where there is waste, there is a duty to stop it escaping. It should be stored safely and securely. When handing on the

waste to someone else, secure it in a suitable container. Loose material in a skip or a vehicle should be covered. Check that the person taking the waste away is legally authorized to do so. The persons allowed to take away waste are:

Council Waste Collectors. For most shops and small offices, the council will collect the waste. In this case no more checking will be needed (there will be some paperwork).
Registered Waste Carriers. Carriers of waste have to be registered with the council. Look at the carrier's certificate of registration.
Exempt Waste Carriers. Not all carriers will be registered, for example charities and voluntary organizations. If they say they are exempt, ask them why.
Holders of Waste Material or Waste Management Licences. Some licences are only valid for certain types of waste or certain activities. Checks should be made to see if they cover the type of waste being taken away.

Persons who are exempt from the requirement to have waste disposal or waste management licences. There are exemptions for very specific activities and types of waste. If someone claims not to need a licence, a check should be made for the exemptions in their case.

Paper Work
When waste changes hand, a transfer note must be completed and signed by both parties and a written description of the waste handed over. These two pieces of information may be on a single piece of paper. The Government has produced a model form, but any forms may be used provided they contain the right kind of information. Repeated transfers of the same kind of waste between the same parties can be covered by one transfer note for up to one year, e.g. weekly collections by the council from one shop.

Transfer Note
This must include:

What the waste is and how much there is.

What sort of container it is in.
The time and date the waste was transferred.
Where the transfer took place.
The names and the addresses of both parties.
Details of the category of each authorized person.
Whether either or both parties, as a waste carrier, has a registration certificate.
The certificate number and the name of the council that issued it. If either or both of the parties has a waste licence, the transfer note must include the licence number of the council that issued it.
Reasons for any exemptions from the requirement to register or have a licence.

The written description must provide as much information as possible, since someone else might need to handle the waste safely.

Both parties must keep copies of the transfer note and the description for two years. They may have to prove in court where the waste came from and what they did with it. Action should be taken if it is suspected that someone else is dealing with waste illegally, before or after reaching the destination.

DO NOT give waste to or take waste from any party suspected of dealing waste illegally. Report immediately to the council if suspicious.
DO remember that bacteria multiply rapidly in refuse and waste food.
DO separate waste food from fresh food and dispose of it.
DO ensure staff wash their hands after handling waste.
DO store waste securely and safely and check the paperwork.

3 Staff

FOOD HANDLERS

A food handler, by definition, is anyone working where food is stored, prepared, cooked, served, displayed or sold. The regulations relate directly to virtually anyone working in food premises. The responsibilities are directly those of the food handler, who can be taken to court for offences against the regulations. Any proprietor or manager must ensure that the people they employ as food handlers must comply with these regulations as they can be liable to prosecution under regulation 29. Food handlers have a number of responsibilities under regulations 9, 10, 11, 12 and 13. The food handler is responsible for ensuring that bacteria are not allowed the conditions for growth and for preventing them growing to sufficient numbers in food to cause food poisoning. They must ensure the correct storage and thorough cooking of the food they are handling. They must maintain high standards of personal hygiene and be aware of all the possible sources of contamination in the kitchen.

The food handler can contaminate the food by way of bacteria that are present in the human body and by cross contamination. Food handlers should ensure that the food handling area is clean and that the equipment and utensils they are using are clean and in good repair.

DO ensure that employees undergo a basic food hygiene course, so that they are aware of the problems that food handlers can cause.

When selecting staff as food handlers, prospective employees should be in good health and be aware of the need for high standards of food hygiene. Potential employees who do not take the trouble to present a good appearance at interview are not likely to achieve the high standard of hygiene you will require. Previous knowledge should be an advantage, particularly a formal hygiene qualification. Poorly presented staff may lead to a loss in customers, reputation and profits.

Some companies now insist on routine medical and laboratory screening of food handlers before employment is offered. This consists of providing a sample of faeces for laboratory bacteriological examination, to ensure that the potential employee has no infection. There is no evidence that routinely screening employees in this manner will be of much benefit to your business, but a pre-employment questionnaire should be completed by potential employees, and a health questionnaire should be routinely completed. You will need these records to prove the defence of 'due dilligence'. Have the questionnaire screened by a doctor, who, if concerned, can follow it up.

If you supply food to countries within the EC, all caterers are obliged to screen all food handlers on a regular basis.

Food handlers are required by law to notify their employers if they suspect they are suffering the symptoms of food poisoning, septic cuts and boils or any staphylococcus infections and nose or throat infections. The employer is then required to inform Environmental Health. A boil is a tender, raised, pus-filled area on the skin and is caused by the bacteria staphylococcus aureus. The bacteria enter the skin through a hair follicle or sweat gland, or through a scratch or other break in the skin. Boils will contain millions of staphylococcus aureus.

TRAINING

Food hygiene is a management issue and, with the introduction of the Food Safety Act, the legislation has been designed to make management take responsibility for food hygiene.

The background to the training issue is that as early as July 1989 the Government earmarked training as a priority. In the White Paper *Food Safety – Protecting the Consumer* it was stated that provision would be made for the compulsory training of 'those people who handle food directly'. In 1989 a consultation document was issued, and in June 1990 this period of consultation ended. Meanwhile the Food Safety Act came into force and food authorities were 'authorized to provide training courses in food hygiene' and ministers were 'empowered' to make regulations 'secure in the observance of hygiene'. Draft regulations are still awaited, but it is worth emphasizing that, under the Food Safety Act, enforcement officers may at any time issue an improvement notice requiring training to be carried out in a stated period. More importantly, it is certain that training records will be crucial to a business trying to prove 'due dilligence' in court.

Who should train? The training market is bursting at the seams with people who see an opportunity for making money by issuing a maximum number of certificates at discount prices. I have even been offered money to issue the certificates without teaching the course! These people are not trainers or concerned with the effects of training staff to a required standard. Training is a skilled profession so check the qualifications of the people teaching your staff. All trainers should have formal qualifications from either The Royal Institute of Environmental Health Offices, The Royal Institute of Public Health and Hygiene or The Royal Society of Health. Colleges running courses may well be an option for some businesses to train their own trainers by investing in advanced food hygiene managers. Training is thus kept in-house, a cost effective option since cascade training (one qualified staff member teaching others) is then possible. In-house training can be more appropriate to the work place.

CARRIERS

A small percentage of the population are carriers of pathogenic bacteria. Although they do not have any of the symptoms of food poisoning, pathogenic bacteria are present in their intestines and therefore their faeces. Convalescent carriers are people who have had food poisoning recently, although they are fit and healthy and fully recovered they will carry the pathogenic bacteria in their faeces. Healthy carriers are people who have not suffered the symptoms of food poisoning, but carry pathogenic bacteria in their intestines and will pass the bacteria in their faeces. Both convalescent and healthy carriers run the risk of contaminating their hands with food poisoning bacteria when they visit the toilet, so thorough cleaning of the hands must be ensured after visiting the toilet. Convalescent carriers will know they are high risks as food handlers, and should be placed on non-food duties until they have stopped passing the bacteria.

A communicable disease is a disease which is transmitted from one person to another, or from an animal to a person. It may or may not be contagious, that is caught by touching objects that an infected person has handled, or through direct contact with him. Communicable diseases include common cold, flu and cholera. They are sometimes transmitted by carriers. Faecal oral contamination is where pathogenic bacteria from food handlers will be excreted when visiting the toilet. Soft toilet tissue will allow the bacteria to pass on to the hands, and, if the hands are not washed thoroughly, the next food the food handler touches will become contaminated. Thus, food that has been contaminated in this way has been contaminated by the faecal oral route.

HAIR

To comply with regulation 9 (Food to be Protected from Risk of Contamination) and regulation 11 (Overclothing) hair must be kept covered by food handlers. Hair may contain staphylococcus aureus. The following is a quote from a recent (April 1992) report by an EHO on a small shop where food is prepared, cooked and served. Four members of staff are employed and all are involved in all aspects of the catering tasks.

'There is a tendency for the current fashion in hairstyles to be grown long and bunched or left loose. I am concerned that such styles in particular may give rise to persons touching their hair. There is also a contamination risk should hair fall out. I would consider it reasonable that a suitable hairnet or similar be used by all food handlers working in the shop to comply with Regulations 9 and 11.'

Hair is constantly falling out and contains bacteria. Any hair falling into food should not be tolerated. Hair should be kept clean and a suitable hair covering should be worn that prevents hair falling into food.

DO NOT forget that the only suitable hair covering is a hair net.

Hair and head coverings should be adjusted away from the food area.

HANDS

Food poisoning bacteria carried on the hands and transferred on to food during its preparation is one of the most common causes of food poisoning. Bacteria in the faeces can be transferred through soft toilet tissue and on to the hands after visiting the toilet and so on to food. Staphylococcus present on staff can be transferred to hands by blowing the nose, dipping fingers into foods to taste, licking fingers to separate bags. Smoking a cigarette will transfer bacteria from the mouth to the hands. Washing hands after all of these will rid the hands of bacteria. Salmonella bacteria will be transferred to the hands after preparing raw poultry. Septic cuts on the hands will contain millions of staphylococcus aureus. There are several ways of looking after your hands:

DO keep fingernails short, and clean them with a nail-brush.
DO NOT wear nail varnish. It chips, it flakes, and it will fall into food. Food handlers have a tendency to put their fingers in their mouths to scratch off the nail varnish.
DO NOT wear jewellery. The skin underneath the rings will harbour a large number of bacteria especially if the rings are not removed when the hands are being washed.
DO NOT bite fingernails. This will transfer bacteria from the mouth to the hands.
DO cover cuts and sores with a waterproof dressing of a distinctive colour. Any person with a septic cut, boil or whitlow should be taken off food duties.
DO keep hands clean.
DO pay attention to cross contamination and wash hands after handling raw meat and poultry.

DO NOT handle food excessively. Use something else, tongs, spoon etc.

Hand Washing

Normal hand washing, even when done properly, is likely to leave surprisingly large numbers of bacteria on the hands. This may be dangerous for food handlers. Such is the structure of the skin, that absolute sterility is impossible to achieve by chemical or any other means, without destruction of the skin itself. However, good results can be obtained by using the following techniques:

Using a bactericidal washing cream or soap. These preparations are widely used in hospitals where sterility of the hands is very important. They are supplied in containers which slide into a wall mounted dispenser. The active anti-bacterial agent is usually hexachlorophane; the soap should be non-perfumed.

Use of a barrier cream after washing. The main function of an antiseptic barrier cream is to reduce the numbers of bacteria left on the skin after washing and provide an invisible odourless film on the hands, which will prevent the transfer of pathogenic organisms. It is not a substitute for proper hand washing and should not be used as a washing cream. Barrier creams contain fats and other substances which replace the natural oils of the skin lost through constant contact with water and prevent chaffing of the hands. The active anti-bacterial agent is hexachlorophane or bengalkonium chloride.

Antiseptic inhibits growth but does not kill bacteria.

Germicide, sterilant or disinfectant kills bacteria.

Deodorant absorbs or corrects odour but does not kill bacteria.

DO wash hands before handling food, after cleaning, after visiting the toilet, after touching hair, face, nose or mouth, after coughing or sneezing, after smoking, after handling raw meat and poultry.

Hand Drying

By far the best method for drying hands is an electric, automatic hot air dryer. Any bacteria left on the hands after washing will not be transferred anywhere else. It should be sited above or next to the washhand basin. One possible disadvantage is the time a dryer takes to dry the hands; staff in a busy kitchen may be tempted to finish drying their hands on their clothing or cloths.

Disposable paper towels are suitable and cheap, the paper should be used once and then disposed of. They should be in a dispenser and fixed to the wall for easy availability. A suitable covered bin should be sited for the used paper.

If roller towels are used they should be provided by a commercial laundry contract to ensure they are changed daily. Not having facilities for drying hands is an offence under regulation 18.

DO NOT use towelling as a method for drying hands.
DO NOT allow chefs or cooks to carry a cloth tucked into their aprons to wipe their hands on or to wipe knives on.

A recent outbreak of food poisoning at a catering college was puzzling at first. All the students who were taken ill had not eaten meat just salads. It was discovered the chef had prepared raw chicken to make chicken pies and had used the cloth hanging from his apron to wipe both his hands and his knives. He then prepared the salads. He transferred the bacteria from his hands and knives to the salads. None of the people who had eaten the cooked chicken were taken ill.

Perfume should not be worn by a food handler. The smell may taint the food, and sometimes the perfume is worn to mask poor personal hygiene of the wearer. The practice of wearing perfume should be discouraged.

The wearing of jewellery should also be discouraged. A food handler should not wear earrings, necklaces, watches, bracelets or rings. Whereas the food handler may be aware of a good handwashing routine, the skin in contact with jewellery particularly rings will not be thoroughly clean. Underneath the rings will provide the ideal conditions for bacterial growth, especially if the food handler is involved in several tasks in the food preparation area, handling raw meat and poultry then jobs involving other foods. Ornate or loose-fitting jewellery should not be permitted because of the risk of cross contamination and the fact that it can be a safety hazard when handling knives or using machinery.

DO permit only a plain gold wedding band to be worn. It can be covered with a detectable waterproof dressing.

A high standard of personal hygiene must be demanded of all food handlers. They should be encouraged to bath or shower regularly, to keep as clean as possible when working in the kitchen, and to avoid bad habits which could encourage the spread of bacteria. Hands come into direct contact with food and must be kept clean at all times. They should only be washed in a washhand basin with an unperfumed germicidal liquid soap. A nail-brush must be used to thoroughly clean the nails. Dry thoroughly using a hot air dryer or paper towels. The hands should be washed on entering the food preparation area, before handling food, after handling raw meat, using the toilet, removing waste and rubbish, blowing the nose, touching the hair and face, smoking and cleaning duties and whenever they may have been contaminated.

DO NOT touch the nose, mouth and ears in the food area.
DO NOT smoke in the food area.
DO NOT allow the food handlers to eat sweets or chew gum in the food area.
DO insist on clean protective clothing being worn in the food area and on the removal of outdoor clothing and personal belongings to somewhere outside the food handling area.
DO set up a reporting procedure for staff to inform you if they are ill, especially for a gastrointestinal illness, septic cuts and boils or any infection of the nose, mouth and throat.

The bacteria staphylococcus aureus is present on some 50% of the population and the other 50% will pick it up during the day. It will be present in the nose, mouth and ears, and touching these will increase the risk of cross contamination by transferring the bacteria from these parts of the body to food.

Sneezing is an involuntary reflex action to remove irritation from the nasal passages. The irritation may be temporary from inhaling dust, pepper or snuff, or it may be caused by inflamation from the common cold, hayfever and some types of asthma.

When a person sneezes due to a cold he sprays a cloud of infectious droplets several feet through the air unless he sneezes into a handkerchief. Sneezing is one of the principal ways such diseases are spread. The bacteria present is staphylococcus aureus.

Disposable tissue should be used for blowing the nose. The tissue should be disposed of and the hands thoroughly washed. Food handlers with a heavy cold should be put on non-food duties to avoid coughing and sneezing in the food preparation area. Bacteria can be spread over a wide area in droplets of water from coughing and sneezing.

DO NOT allow staff to handle food if they have a heavy cold.
DO NOT employ staff who obviously bite their nails since their fingers will be constantly in their mouths.

Bar staff in pubs are classed as food handlers if they handle meals and snacks. If they only handle and serve drinks and packaged goods, e.g. nuts and crisps they are exempt from regulation 11 (Protective Clothing).

Drink is classified as food and is subject to the Food Safety Act 1990 and the Food Hygiene Regulations 1970. Bar staff should pay particular attention to the cleanliness of glasses and should check that they are visibly clean before they serve the drink. Lipstick remains on a glass may contain staphylococcus aureus, and a white deposit on the inside of the glass could mean that the chemicals used for cleaning in a dishwasher/glass washer is at the wrong strength.

Smoking in a food room is illegal. The fine is now up to £2,000, and this includes the back of a bar. Apart from the obvious problems caused by cigarette ash falling into food or drink, cigarettes need to be put out somewhere, and cigarette ends may eventually find their way into food either deliberately or accidentally. Smoke can taint the food and make it unpleasant to eat. A not so obvious problem is that smokers contaminate their hands by touching their mouths when they smoke. Staphylococcus aureus bacteria present in the mouth will be transferred to the hands.

Smokers frequently have coughs associated with smoking so they are likely to cough more than people who do not smoke. If you employ smokers as food handlers you should provide somewhere for them to smoke on their breaks. Otherwise they will use nearby toilets or open doorways, and tend to extinguish half-smoked cigarettes, put them into their pockets and then bring them into the food room.

DO NOT allow smoking anywhere near the food room.
DO NOT allow smoking in the staff toilets.
DO insist on hands being washed when returning from a break.

4 Hazards

ANIMALS

Animals as a source of infection to man may be diseased or simply carriers. Many animals transmit diseases to man including cats, dogs, cattle, pigs and rodents. Among the diseases they transmit are tuberculosis (cows, from milk), brucellosis (cows, from milk), rabies (dogs), salmonella infections (rodents, birds, cattle etc.), plague (rats), tapeworms (pigs and cattle), leptospiral jaundice (rats) and trichinosis (pigs).

Animal Reservoirs of Salmonella Organisms
These include:

Horses, cattle, pigs, ducks, chickens, mice, rats, birds, terrapins, turkeys, cats, dogs, frogs, snakes and any other domestic animals.
Meat for pets and humans, offal, eggs, egg products and poultry, raw milk and excreta.

The term vector is applied to any living carrier of an infectious disease but is usually limited to insects and animals that transmit such diseases in various ways to human beings. For instance, houseflies may carry food poisoning bacteria and typhoid bacteria and deposit them on food.

PEST CONTROL

Pest control is absolutely vital for any business, especially if the business is a food business where food is manufactured, packed, prepared or served. Pests are particularly attracted to the kinds of conditions found in a hotel, restaurant or canteen kitchen. A wide variety of insects, mites and some species of birds and animals enter food premises because they know they will find food, warmth and shelter there.

Food

Even in small quantities food enables pests to thrive and breed.

Warmth

Pests of all types are attracted to buildings which offer even a limited amount of warmth. These conditions will provide the conditions for breeding.

Shelter

Any building will provide the ideal shelter for pests. Modern buildings with suspended ceilings, cavity walls (sometimes insulated with corrugated cardboard), service ducts and enclosed electrical trunking are more likely to create a pest risk than older buildings without these features. Avoid boxing in pipes.

Many organisms can lead to illness for the consumer and loss of production reputation for the caterer.

Pests are prohibited by legislation. Owners of premises have a legal responsibility to exclude pests from their premises. They cause expensive deterioration, spread dangerous bacteria and could destroy the reputation of any catering establishment.

Many pests are carriers of disease. Mice leave sixty to eighty droppings and urine droplets wherever they move. Mice urine has bacteria that cause disease; their droppings contain pathogens including those of the salmonella group. Flies, cockroaches and ants will leave excretory deposits and vomit.

It should be emphasized that clean, well constructed and well maintained premises will not show signs of pests. Always be on the lookout for the following signs:

Live or dead birds, insect or rodent carcasses.
Droppings.
Torn sacks or bags.
Holes in cardboard boxes or containers.

Food handlers should be constantly on the lookout for pests and maintain high standards of food hygiene to discourage them. Any signs of infestation should be reported so that a suitable pest control can be undertaken.

In a recently reported case of prosecution for breaking food hygiene by a city council a restaurant owner admitted seventeen charges. The court was told that a decomposed rat carcass was found under a food display cabinet, rat droppings were found and also the remains of a rats' nest. He was fined £7,000 with £170 costs. At the same time another restaurant owner admitted twenty charges which included cockroaches under a refrigerator, larder beetles and a fly pupae in a food preparation room and rat droppings. He was fined £3,200 with £777 costs.

There is a legal duty under the Prevention of Pests Act 1949 and the Food Hygiene Regulations 1970 to keep premises free from infestation and to report an infestation to local authorities. In addition all pesticides and the method of use must comply with the requirements for the Control of Substances Hazardous to Health (COSHH) Regulations 1988. There are three lines of pest control that you can take: exclusion, restriction and destruction.

Exclusion
Wherever possible keep pests out, keep your building structure sound, no broken air bricks, no gaps under doors or around windows, keep outside walls clear of rubbish or weeds. Check skirting-boards and fill any gaps around work units (using a proprietary filler). Check around pipes bringing in water and gas, any gaps should be filled in to stop rodents and insects gaining access. Strip curtains on outside doors in warehouses and dispatch bays will help to prevent

birds and flying insects getting in.

Restriction

Restriction means denying pests access, a safe place to live. Preventive measures include thorough cleaning, removing waste throughout the working day, sealing holes where pipes pass through interior walls, good stock rotation and correct storage of food materials. When checking goods in, check for signs of pests.

Destruction

If, despite all your efforts, you discover you have a pest problem, chemical pesticides may be required. Because of the risk involved in administering chemicals (if any pesticides or chemicals come into contact with food, chemical food poisoning may result), the use of such chemicals must be stricly controlled. The best control is to seek expert advice and call in a pest control company. Try your local Environmental Health Office, who will provide a limited service for free or for a modest charge. Companies who are members of the British Pest Control Association (BPCA) will be able to identify and trace the extent of the infestation and select the best method for the treatment of the problem.

Mice and Rats

Because of their different biology and behaviour a variety of control methods are used. Ready to use rodenticide baits for mice and rats include bromadiolene, brodifacoum and difencom; other baits for mice include calciserol and alphachloralose. Certain rodenticidal gels or contact dust can be pumped into wall and floor cavities so that the pest will lick it off when cleaning their fur and feet.

Flies

Fit fly screens on opening windows. Fly sprays using pyrethrin or pyrethrin-based should not be used in food preparation areas, over open or exposed food.

DO NOT use fly strips which give off an insecticidal vapour that may taint the food. The best method, and that commonly fitted in food rooms, is the ultraviolet electrical fly killing device. The following guidelines should be followed.

Staff safety should be considered. Bearing in mind the fact that these units operate on a high voltage current, and that the natural flight path for a fly is two metres or under, the units need to be sited correctly to be effective. The unit should be sited no more than 2.6 metres from the floor and wherever possible at a right angle to a natural light source.

Position units away from doorways and open windows; draughts and strong currents mean there is a risk that dead insects will be blown out of the collection tray on to the food area.

Insects are strongly attracted by the smell of food, so site units close to where the food smell is strongest.

Site units away from natural sunlight since this will maximize the lure of ultraviolent. The tubes should be replaced every twelve months. Even though the tubes will light up, the coating may have deteriorated and become less than 100% effective.

Make sure that the killing grid is specified, or it may not have enough power to kill on contact, or trap insects on the bars causing unnecessary electrical charges.

Check that the unit is safe and conforms to British Standards.

Wasps

Call in the experts to deal with a nest located on or near your premises. If the premises are in an isolated position a perimeter bait is available that has a slow acting insecticide; the workers take this back to the nest and thus eliminate the colony. Small numbers of wasps can be dealt with like flies.

Moths

If moths are a problem, thoroughly clean all machinery, storage areas and surfaces before treatment. Long lasting sprays of fenitrothian or iodofinphos may be applied to walls, ceilings, shelves and racks. Pheremone traps which attract moths can be used on certain moth species. Clothes'-moths and house moths can be destroyed by spraying with a good moth proofer, after thorough cleaning.

Ants

Baiting with raw liver is often used to get the ants to reveal their nests and baits containing methopreme or boric acid are an effective control method.

Cockroaches

For successful control of crawling insects you have to take the insecticide to the insect, and this should only be done by the specialists. It requires specialist spraying equipment, using chemicals in spray or powder form. Various methods are used to meet the different demands of different premises under infestation. Some of the effective forms of insecticide in use at present are iodofephos, alphacypermethin and bendiocarb.

It must be emphasized that these should only be administered by the experts and specialized advice always sought. It has become increasingly difficult to eliminate insects in modern buildings or buildings that have been renovated. Panelled walls, boxed in pipes, concealed lighting, false ceilings and cavity walls, soundproofed or insulated with corrugated cardboard, all provide insects with a safe undisturbed place to live.

Birds

Polythene netting can be used as a barrier to keep birds from nesting in alcoves, roof voids, guttering etc. Another method, where birds have become a serious problem, is the avistrand system of plastic-covered wires kept tight by steel springs fixed to buildings. If birds are considered to be a health hazard or damage is being caused inside premises, they can be removed by obtaining a licence from MAFF to use a bait containing the drug alphachloralose which renders the bird unconscious. The bird is then collected and humanely killed. This method ensures any protected bird that takes the bait can recover and be returned to the wild. Selected shooting by a skilled marksman with specially designed rifles is another option, and pigeons can be live trapped by cage traps.

Pets

Pets should be put in the same category as pests, as they are likely to come into contact with food poisoning bacteria by the places they visit or through the food that they eat. Pet food is usually heavily contaminated with bacteria, so separate utensils and equipment must be used for opening and removing food from the cans and for the pets to eat from.

PESTS

Rats

Rats and mice have fast growing incisor teeth with which they gnaw hard materials to keep their teeth at the right length and razor sharp. Packaging, wooden doors, gas and water pipes, electric cables and plastic fittings are damaged, sometimes with disastrous results, e.g. fires can start by electric cables being stipped of their PVC insulation.

Rats frequently carry salmonella in their intestines so their droppings will contain live bacteria. They carry bacteria on their fur and feet and will transfer bacteria from soil, waste food, drains, sewers and refuse to uncovered food and work surfaces for food preparation just by travelling over them. Rats' urine sometimes carries leptospiral icterohaemorrhagie which causes Weil's disease. The bacteria enters the body through cuts and abrasions on the skin or through the mucus membranes of the nose, mouth or eyes.

DO ensure that the food handler covers all cuts and sores on their hands.

Rats live and breed in warm, dark corners where they will not be disturbed. They are creatures of habit and will follow defined paths to and from foods, usually keeping close to walls and pipes to avoid open spaces.

A typical brown rat weighs approximately 0.5 kg and a breeding pair will produce 3-6 litters a year, each litter containing about 10 young; 200 rats can develop in a year and with favourable conditions a pair and their young can increase to 2,000. Their droppings are spindle-shaped and their dark fur has a greasy substance in it that will be left behind when they move close to walls; it may be the first indication that is noticed. Footprints in flour or dust are another indication that rats are present. Storerooms should be thoroughly cleaned, all stock kept off the floor and rotated to ensure rats are not sheltering at the back of the room.

DO check for signs of nibbled packets or sacks of food, footprints in spilt flour, hairs on food or equipment. There will also be a characteristic smell on contaminated food. Check for greasy marks left on walls and surfaces, droppings on the floor or gnaw marks.

Mice

Mice are erratic, sporadic feeders, which means they can be difficult to catch and will nibble at a variety of foods. They can exist for long periods on just the moisture from their food supply. An adult mouse can exist on just 3 grammes a day.

They will leave 60–80 droppings per day and innumerable urine droplets wherever they travel. Mice droppings will contain salmonella which are easily transmitted on to surfaces and food over which they travel, often at night. They show an erratic pattern of movement, feeding from 200 different points in the night. They can scale sheer vertical walls and pipes and squeeze through tiny gaps; they have no defined paths or routes.

Mice are very prolific breeders having ten litters a year of up to sixteen young, so the infestation problem can become very serious in a short period of time.

DO remember prevention is better than cure.
DO train staff to search for pests regularly and to recognize any signs of any infestation.
DO routinely move and clean behind large pieces of equipment.
DO NOT permit a safe quiet environment for pests.
DO NOT attempt to deal with an infestation problem yourself, contact a specialist pest control company and keep records for due diligence.

An example of a recent prosecution:

Environmental Health Officers visited a mini market following a number of complaints. Magistrates were told that while one officer was waiting in the shop a mouse ran out.

The inspectors found the shop was overrun with mice. There were mice droppings on window sills, under shelves and in the food store of the mini market. Apart from the mice, they found dirty shelves, ripped carpet and grease and dirt around the freezer. An old apple core, decomposing, was found under one of the shelves. In defence the court was told 'the owner began the business in 1989 and found it more than she could handle. She was a mother of three, running a shop and caring for her home and family. The shop backed on to open land and the entire road had been plagued by mice, and the mice had proved difficult to eradicate.' She had since followed advice from the Environmental Health Department and no problem now existed. She pleaded guilty to four breaches of the Food Safety Act and was fined £600 and ordered to pay £260 costs.

Another example:

A Chinese take-away had to be closed down, after layers of dirt and mouse droppings were found by inspectors in cooking and storage areas. The droppings were discovered around bags of rice stored on a wooden pallet at the take-away. Droppings were also found on a unit containing a box of raw red meat. A gap at the bottom of the door allowed mice to infest the storage shed. Cooked chickens were left uncovered at room temperature and ingrained dirt and grease caked the floors and ceiling in the cooking area. They pleaded guilty to fourteen charges concerning insanitary conditions at their Chinese take-away. The Environmental Health Officers visited the premises after the owners contacted the borough council's pest control department to report their mice problem. The officer immediately applied for an Emergency Prohibition Order and the couple were served with several improvement notices. The couple were fined £700 and ordered to pay £150 costs.

Flies

The most common housefly (musca domestica) and the blowfly (calliophora vomitoria) are the most dangerous insect pests that inhabit catering premises. Flies tend to be tolerated in food premises, but their danger to health should not be underestimated. Flies feed on waste food, dirt and refuse from which they fly to human food, where they deposit bacteria from their wings, legs, saliva and excrement. They are capable of spreading food poisoning bacteria, dysentery and typhoid.

Flies breed very rapidly, laying their eggs in waste material, dustbins, waste food and uncovered food. Five or six batches of eggs are laid in a season, with 120–150 eggs in each batch. In summer temperatures it takes only twelve hours for the eggs to hatch and develop into maggots.

Bluebottles are attracted to meat and fish products on which they lay their eggs. All species of flies feed by vomiting their saliva on to the food surface, treading it in and sucking up the resulting liquid. In the course of doing this the fly will contaminate the food with bacteria from the gut and feet. Flies defecate while feeding and their faeces carry salmonella, other pathogenic organisms and the eggs of parasitic worms.

DO remove places where flies are likely to lay their eggs, rubbish and tips should not be near buildings where food is being prepared or stored.
DO have tight-fitting lids on dustbins.
DO NOT allow staff to open windows for ventilation without first fitting fly screens.

Cockroaches

There are two types of cockroach found in the UK: the German cockroach (blattells germanica) and the Oriental cockroach (blatta orientalis). Despite fifty years of pest control operations against them, they are two of the most widely distributed pests of the catering industry. Hotel and restaurant kitchens, and bars all provide warm, humid and safe hiding-places.

The German cockroach likes warmth and often chooses to live and breed behind ovens, hot water pipes and refrigeration motors. The Oriental cockroach prefers a damper, cooler environment, like a cellar or warehouse.

Regular inspections must be carried out, even if you are sure you do not have the insect on the premises, as the egg capsule can be introduced to the premises by way of a flour sack or beer crate. Many cockroaches have developed resistance to certain insecticides, so if these insects are suspected on the premises, seek expert advice. Most premises will afford entry to cockroaches, as they can squeeze through the narrowest gaps and crevices. If they are spotted during daylight hours, the chances are that there is an infestation problem, because they will only normally come out at night in search of food. They will contaminate food and the surfaces they crawl over. They carry salmonella bacteria and will contaminate more food than they eat. They like drains, sewers and rubbish and an infestation is characterised by a very unpleasant 'tomcat' smell.

The female will not make a nest to lay her eggs, preferring instead to lay then wherever she is; she could be crawling up a kitchen wall when she lays them. The young when they hatch out are almost colourless, but turn a light brown colour after a few days. There is a progressive darkening of colour to a dark brown. The male will grow to about 12 mm and is then too large to stay on the wall and will fall back to the floor. Effective pest control will kill the female and adult species, usually by spraying infected areas or taping cockroach traps to known runs. Several treatments will be necessary as the eggs are protected by a capsule and do not hatch out for several months.

DO train staff so that they can check whether pests are likely to be found.
DO know the signs of infestation.
DO understand why cleaning is so important.
DO realize that all pests are looking for warmth, food and shelter.

Moths

There are several millmoths and commodity moths that find their way into catering ingredients:

Warehouse moth (ephestia elutella). The grub feeds on cocoa beans, chocolate products, nuts and flour. The larvae produce silky webbing, which in any quantity can restrict the ventilation of ingredients stored in sacks or bags. The adult is an active flier covering large areas.

The Indian meal moth (plodia interpunctella) often forms

its white cocoon in the folds of wrapping paper, cardboard cartons or cake boxes, and if these are not available the plodia grubs often hide in crevices in the actual building structure.

Tropical warehouse moth (cadra cantella) normally pupates close to its food.

Both cadra and plodia attack fruit and nuts, cereal and chocolate products. Both can be brought into a larder or dry food store in consignments of dried fruits. The adults of both species are most active between May and August. The grubs emerge and move about in late summer to early autumn.

DO check regularly for any signs of this infestation.
DO keep records of pest control.

Beetles

There are a number of beetles that can cause a problem on food premises. Many species can survive on food debris in cracks and crevices, particularly the bread or biscuit beetle.

Bread beetles complete their life-cycle in seven months and the grub survives starvation for a week. The short life-cycle means it is most important to use the correct insecticide to be sure of clearing up the infestation.

Hide beetles, spider beetles and larder beetles are attracted by meat and protein products. The flour beetle is now a major pest of flour, and they multiply rapidly. Flour that becomes infested with the flour beetle smells sour and becomes useless for making bread as it will not rise satisfactorily.

Other dried ingredients are prone to infestation by the flour mite and spider beetle. The most common spider beetle is the Australian spider beetle. These are not major pests like the flour beetle but they will thrive in any cereal waste, such as spilt flour, scraps of dough and other food materials. The flour beetle is small in size and will not be noticed until there is a major infestation. They will exist in food stores and kitchens and will infest fresh consignments of food stuffs as they arrive on premises. A typical spider beetle has a round shaped body, is about 3 mm long and has long legs in comparison to its body. It feeds on cereal residues, dried fruit debris and animal remains. The adult avoids light and likes a damp atmosphere, with plenty of moisture. It lays up to a hundred eggs a time, from which emerge a whitish fleshy grub. The pupa forms a tough, spherical cocoon and the complete life cycle takes three months.

DO destroy any infected food.
DO clean the store thoroughly.
DO use a pest control company to treat the area and deter reinfestation.
DO use a pest control recording system and keep the records to prove due dilligence.

In a recent court case heard in the Midlands, the proprietor of a bakery shop was fined £900 with £165 costs for three offences including carrying on a business in insanitary conditions. Flour mites were found in a flour bag, larder beetles were present on the premises, dirty trays under the refrigerators and food waste under equipment.

Birds

You have a legal responsibility under the Food Hygiene (Amended) Regulations 1989 'to prevent so far as reasonably possible, entry of birds and any risk of infestation by rats, mice or insects'.

Birds have been a source of food poisoning outbreaks. Both salmonella and campylobacter have been identified in their droppings. Birds such as sparrows, pigeons and starlings should not be allowed access to food premises since their nests and droppings encourage the breeding of parasites, pests and stored product insects. Their feathers are infested with insects and mites, and if they get into food stores they can be very difficult to remove.

In cash and carrys and warehouses birds can become a real pest, often nesting high up in the roof and coming down to feed, damaging sacks of flour etc. The droppings can damage the actual fabric of the building through fungi growing on the droppings creating acids which eat into the stone or brick work.

DO NOT allow birds access, fit ventilation grids or wire grids on windows which open. Stop birds perching on eaves or guttering.

DO NOT allow staff to feed birds since this encourages them to stay.

Ants

Garden ants can become a problem in catering premises. They live outdoors and will nest in cracked paving, under stones, under plant roots and tree stumps. Ants have a very acute sense of smell and will quickly find and infest exposed food of all kinds. Worker ants will enter buildings in search of sweet foods. Flying ants are the winged reproductive ants, emerging from the nest for a few days in the summer. Pharaoh's ants (monomorium pharaonis) were introduced to this country 100 years ago from the Middle East and are now established as a common pest. They are usually found in centrally heated buildings. Each nest may contain up to 5,000 ants including 100 queens, each of whom lays approximately twelve eggs per day. Ants transmit disease and vomit and excrete on everything they come into contact with. The nuisance of ants in food premises can lose business, customers and staff.

Wasps

There is no evidence to suggest that wasps are implicated in the spreading of disease, but they are a nuisance. If a wasp nest is located on the premises it should be destroyed.

SOIL

Soil contains spores of clostridium perfringens and clostridium botulinum. Soil commonly harbours disease-producing bacteria. In particular, any wounds on the hands becoming contaminated with soil may result in tetanus or gas gangrene.

DO clean all raw vegetables before preparation.
DO buy from a reputable supplier and choose those vegetables that are not heavily contaminated with soil.
DO NOT allow deliveries of vegetables to be brought through the food preparation area, and DO clean areas, equipment, utensils and surfaces immediately if they have been contaminated by soil.

PLANTS

Many species of plants are poisonous, and parts of otherwise edible plants are poisonous. For example, potato that has been exposed to the light turns green and develops solanin which causes illness or even death if eaten in large quantities. Other plants that can cause food poisoning include the berries of deadly nightshade; laburnum seeds and leaves; rhubarb leaves, which contain toxic amounts of oxalic acid; apricot stones, which contain a substance that can break down in the body to produce cyanide; red kidney beans and haricot beans. The toxin produced can cause acute vomiting and diarrhoea and attacks the red cells of blood, but the toxin is easily killed by boiling for at least fifteen minutes and discarding the water. In 1991 there were 40,000 cases of food poisoning occuring from eating poisonous plants. Unless you know what you are eating, DON'T.

MOULDS AND YEAST

Apart from bacteria, the common micro-organisms found in food are yeast and moulds. Both are responsible for considerable wastage of food in all stages of preparation, but rarely cause food poisoning, although some moulds can produce poisons called mycotoxins, which have caused disease in animals and are suspected for occasionally affecting humans. Some mycotoxins known as aflatoxins have been shown to be capable of causing cancers. Foods are frequently spoiled by moulds, e.g. in grain or nuts stored in damp conditions and the black or blue/green moulds on bread and citrus fruits. Moulds of the penicillin group are used commercially in the production of antibiotics or in the production of certain cheeses.

DO NOT use mouldy foods, throw them away.
DO NOT just scrape off the mouldy part.

Yeast will not cause food poisoning, but food spoilage usually occurs in foods with a high sugar content. Commercial yeasts are used in the production of bread and alcohol.

FUNGI

These are minute plants that do not contain chlorophyl (the green pigment in leafy plants). They may be made of one or many cells. Fungi commonly affect the skin (as in ringworm or thrush), but they may also invade the body internally. A number of species of mushrooms and toadstools are poisonous. The practice of gathering wild fungi should be avoided unless you are an expert on the thousands of mushrooms and toadstools growing wild. Some moulds growing on stored foods are also able to produce poisons called mycotoxins.

CHEMICAL FOOD POISONING

Chemical food poisoning occurs when food is contaminated by chemicals during the growth, preparation, storage or cooking of food. Chemical contamination may taint the food and cause mild to severe illness.

Carelessness in the kitchen is often the cause of this type of food poisoning. Detergents and disinfectants are often bought in bulk or in concentrated form and need to be diluted or decanted into smaller containers. Even when care is taken, spillages and leakages are possible. Such chemicals should be stored away from food and in such a way that they should not spill or leak from their containers, clearly marked and preferably in a cupboard designated 'for chemicals only'. Always label containers and never use empty containers for food storage. There are strict regulations for food producers and manufacturers governing the use of insecticidal sprays, pesticides, food additives and packaging materials.

Several metals found in cooking utensils are poisonous if eaten in sufficient quantities. There is quite a high risk when these metals come into contact with acidic foods; this is one reason why foods should never be left in open cans since the contents may corrode the lining of the can (usually a laquer lining) and make the contents poisonous. There have been outbreaks of zinc poisoning due to the use of galvanized equipment with acid foods.

Chipped enamel pans can cause antimony poisoning,

especially when used for acid foods. Antimony is a highly poisonous semi-metallic element closely resembling arsenic. It was used for making cheap enamelled ware, and has contaminated acid foods when the food was stored in chipped enamel pans.

DO NOT use enamelled pans for catering.

Aluminium

MAFF estimates that the average intake of aluminium is approximately 6 mgms per day; 90% comes from food and the rest from water. The amount of metal picked up from non-coated aluminium saucepans (these will be old pans) is thought to be 0.1 mgm per 100 gm for most foods rising to 0.7 mgm from acid foods, such as stewed apples. With new-coated aluminium pans it is claimed that no aluminium passes from the pans to the food.

DO buy coated pans if purchasing new aluminium pans.
DO NOT use old uncoated pans for cooking acid foods, e.g. fruit.

Cadmium is a poisonous metallic compound resembling zinc. It is used in alloys and paint pigments for some metal-plated utensils and some types of earthenware. In Japan pollution of water flowing on to rice fields has caused cadmium poisoning in people who ate the rice. Victims suffered paralysis and pain and loss of calcium in their bones resulting in deformity, shrinking of the bones and loss of height. Lead poisoning, due to the absorption of lead from water-pipes etc., is a thing of the past, and the use of arsenic as a preservative is strictly controlled by legislation. In recent years the presence of mercury compounds in the flesh of inshore fish has led to the control of estuary waters being polluted by factory waste.

Care must be taken to avoid prolonged contact between acidic foods and equipment containing the metals in the following list:

Aluminium – pots and pans.
Antimony – chipped enamel vessels.
Cadmium – metal-plated utensils and some types of earthenware.

Copper – cooking utensils.
Lead – glazed earthenware.
Zinc – galvanized containers.

The spraying of fruit and vegetables with poisonous insecticides and herbicides increased in the 1970s. It is now more controlled, following investigations by the WHO and the UN which indicated that there was a link between these chemicals (DDT) and liver damage. Fizzy drinks can dissolve dangerous levels of copper from drinks dispensers if the pipes are not regularly flushed through with fresh water. Similar problems have been reported with ice lollies made in copper moulds that had lost their protective tinning. Although chemical food poisoning is quite rare nowadays dramatic incidents have occurred.

In 1965 eighty-four people became ill after eating bread. The bread had been made with flour, which had become contaminated by a chemical hardener or epoxy resin. The hardener had been carried in the same lorry as the flour and spillages of chemical had occured. Chemical poisons are not destroyed by cooking and so the bread remained poisonous.

Most cases of chemical food poisoning fall within the province of home or industrial safety, being caused by carelessly stored chemicals leading to spillages or leakages.

DO NOT use chipped pots and pans.
DO label containers for chemicals with instructions for use.
DO store chemicals away from food, preferably in a clearly marked cupboard.

CROSS CONTAMINATION

Cross contamination is the transfer of bacteria from contaminated foods to uncontaminated food. It is a particular problem when the uncontaminated food will not undergo any further cooking. Cross contamination is frequently caused by the carelessness of the food handler.

DO keep raw meat and poultry separate from cooked meat and poultry.

DO, if you have space, have two refrigerators, one marked raw meat, the other marked cooked meat.
DO, if you do not have such a space, store raw and defrosting meat and poultry at the bottom of the refrigerator so that there is no risk of the juices or blood coming into contact with clean cooked food.
DO identify and separate areas of the kitchen used for the preparation of raw and cooked foods.
DO thoroughly clean and sterilize work surfaces and equipment after use especially after being used for the preparation of raw meat and poultry.
DO keep utensils used for the preparation of raw meat and poultry separate. Use colour coding which helps to reduce the risk of cross contamination by ensuring that the equipment used is for the correct task.
DO wash hands thoroughly. If hands are not washed in between the preparation of different foods (that is, raw and cooked foods), cross contamination will occur.
DO keep the kitchen clean and free from waste food and rubbish.
DO NOT handle foods excessively. Avoid using bare hands, use tongs, spoons etc. instead.

TOXINS

Food poisoning organisms can affect people in two ways:

1 They can enter the body in the food that is eaten and then enter the tissue of the intestine.
2 They can produce waste products that are poisonous.

Such organisms produce toxins in the food itself, and people become ill when they eat the toxins. Organisms that do both include several of the bacillus genus; and there is always the risk of eating poisons (chemicals) that are not related to micro-organisms.

Exotoxin is a poison produced outside bacteria.

Endotoxin is a poison produced inside bacteria and is only released when they die.

Exogenus infection is an infection outside the person infected.

Endogenus infection is an infection within the patient himself.

Organisms producing toxins in the intestines: clostridium perfringens and E. coli.

Organisms producing toxins in the food: staphylococci and botulinum.

Organisms that produce toxins in both the food and the intestines: bacillus cereus.

Other toxins: scombrotoxins, ciguatera, paralytic shellfish poisoning (PSP), fungi, plants and red kidney beans.

Food-borne Infections

Food can become a means of transport for the bacteria. Food-borne diseases are frequently transmitted by contaminated drinking water, by food that has been washed in the water, by shellfish or plants growing in the water, or by drinking dried food mixed with such water. After an earthquake or flooding, drinking water sometimes becomes contaminated with sewage causing large outbreaks of these diseases. The bacteria present do not need time to multiply, so there is no control by storage at the correct temperature. Only a small number of the bacteria needs to be present to cause illness. Some food-borne illnesses are also caused by virus, protozoa or parasitic worms.

Bacterial Food-Borne Diseases	*Viral*
Brucellosis	Amoebic Dysentery
Campylobacter	Cryptosporidium
Cholera	Giardiasis
Dysentry	Hepatitis A
Paratyphoid	Hepatitis B
Typhoid	Non A/Non B Hepatitis
Tuberculosis	Protozoal

Parasitic Worms

Tapeworms

Trichinosis

Tuberculosis is caused by a species of the genus mycobacterium, and it is an infectious, communicable disease. The disease is usually contracted by breathing in the bacteria in droplets of water or by swallowing contaminated food or by drinking unpasteurized milk.

Brucellosis is an infection caused by the bacteria brucella, which usually affects cattle and other livestock. In these animals it is also called undulant fever, Malta fever and mountain fever. It is transmitted to man by contact with an infected animal or its carcass or by drinking unpasteurized infected milk. Butchers and farmers are more likely to contract the disease, and it is rarely passed from person to person. The symptoms of brucellosis are weakness, great exhaustion at the least exertion, headache, general aches and pain, irritability, alternating chills and fever and high sweats. The lymph nodes in the neck and the armpits may be swollen and the spleen enlarged. Without treatment the infection may last for months or even years, but it is rarely fatal. The person who recovers from brucellosis may continue to be irritable and have some degree of mental or emotional disorder. Confirmation of the infection is obtained by growing the bacteria from a sample of the person's blood. Treatment is simple: a vitamin-enriched diet, antibiotics and rest. The recovery rate is very high.

DO NOT use unpasteurized milk from cows or goats.

Ciguatera

This is a contamination of fish, rarely found in fish in the UK but occasionally found in fish from the Caribbean. The fish become contaminated by feeding on toxic algae. The symptoms of this type of food poisoning include numbness of the lips, fingertips and toes shortly after eating, followed by nausea, vomiting and diarrhoea; convulsions and death may follow in rare cases.

Vibrio parahaemolyticus

This is a comma-shaped bacteria that contaminates fish and shellfish in tropical and sub-tropical waters. The few outbreaks that have occured in Great Britain can usually be traced to imported seafood. This bacteria is readily killed by heat. Food that has been contaminated has been found to have been contaminated after cooking because it was left in 'danger zone' conditions and not refrigerated.

Symptoms are abdominal pain and profuse diarrhoea, often with vomiting and fever. The incubation period is twelve to eighteen hours after eating the contaminated food, and the illness lasts from two to five days. Although rare in the UK, vibrio parahaemolyticus is one of the most common causes of food poisoning in Japan. Beware of eating raw fish Japanese style.

Shellfish can be contaminated by typhoid organisms and other faecal types if the layings are in estuaries polluted by sewage outfalls. Mussels can also be contaminated by a toxin produced by dinoflagellates, small sea organisms which live in the mussel. The toxin produced affects the central nervous system. Algal toxins in shellfish produce a form of poisoning known as paralytic shellfish poisoning.

Some shellfish (such as whelks) may contain natural toxins. Such forms of poisoning from shellfish are rare, but since there is no simple way of knowing that seafood is contaminated, you should rely on information on algal blooms in the sea where the shellfish is gathered. Oysters and mussels which feed on tiny sea creatures called dinoflagelattes can cause shellfish paralysis; the toxin paralyses the heart and respiratory muscles. Scombrotoxin is the most important toxin associated with fish. Bacteria growing on certain fish, e.g. tuna, mackerel (particularly smoked mackerel), produce a compound called histamine; symptoms include vomiting, facial flushing, dizzyness, nausea and headaches. The toxin is very heat resistant and canned fish may be contaminated. It is not apparent from the cans that the fish is contaminated so this type of food poisoning is beyond the control of the food handler. However risks can be cut down if fresh or frozen fish is used instead of canned fish.

Cryptosporidium and Giardia Protozoa

The symptoms of being infected are profuse watery diarrhoea which can last for up to two weeks, abdominal pain and fever. Both these protozoa are found in animals including sheep, calves and domestic pets. It can be spread by the person-to-person route, by direct contact with infected farm or pet animals, by swimming in or drinking infected water, or by eating food contaminated by infected water. Sausages, pâté and raw milk have often been reported as causing cryptosporidium infection, and such cases have occured as a result of 'picking' at foods during cooking.

DO insist on good personal hygiene.
DO cook food thoroughly. Normal cooking temperatures for sausages and meat are sufficient to kill the parasite.
DO NOT handle food excessively. Avoid handling food with bare hands.

Giardiasis
Giardiasis is an intestinal disorder caused by infestation with a microscopic parasite, giardia lamblia. It is contracted by eating contaminated food; although the parasite usually produces no symptoms, it sometimes causes diarrhoea. The incubation period is one to four weeks, and the diarrhoea is profuse and watery accompanied by abdominal pain and nausea. The severity of the symptoms vary. Children are less affected than adults, although children are more likely to be affected. The fact that giardiasis is present may only be discovered by accident in microscopical examination of faeces for some other purpose. The condition can be treated with drugs, e.g. mepacrine and metronidazole. The illness occurs worldwide, but is more common in areas of poor sanitation. The main source of infection is the human carrier with direct person-to-person transmission via the faecal-oral route; water and food may also be contaminated.

Protozoa
These are minute one-cell organisms but are larger than bacteria. The main diseases they cause are amoebiaosis resulting in amoebic dysentery and the infection of organs.

Metazoa
These are multicelled parasitic worms. There are three types: flukes, tapeworms and roundworms.

VIRUS
Viruses are much smaller than bacteria. Tiny particles, they can only be seen with an electron microscope. They grow

only in living tissue and cannot grow in food. Viruses need to invade living cells to replicate themselves, but some are able to survive outside cells when conditions are favourable.

Viruses are usually transferred directly from person to person, sometimes in food. Certain infectious viruses which cause vomiting and diarrhoea can be transmitted by water and food, and are subsequently eaten and then spread by the faecal-oral route.

Viruses are preserved by refrigeration and freezing, but are killed by normal cooking processes. They are sensitive to ultraviolet irradiation and disinfection. Infectious viruses which infect through the intestines resist acid conditions and can survive in food such as vinegar. They can also survive in foods containing high levels of sugar and foods preserved in alcohol.

VIRAL CONTAMINATION

This happens in two ways: primary contamination where food is contaminated at source in its growing environment, e.g. shellfish in sewage-contaminated water; and secondary contamination by infected food handlers whilst preparing food.

Primary Contamination at Source

Shellfish: The proof that viruses may be transmitted through food has come from outbreaks of viral illnesses associated with shellfish (molluscs). Most illnesses associated with molluscs are viral not bacterial. Some reported outbreaks have involved hundreds of people. Bivalve molluscs include oysters, clams, mussels and cockles and are traditionally harvested from shallow and inshore waters, but are liable to sewage pollution. Bivalves filter matter (including bacteria and virus) out of the water by passing over their gills. Viruses will not multiply in shellfish, but they can accumulate in large numbers to cause human illness. Shellfish such as cockles are cooked briefly before they are sold, and if cooked for longer periods they become tough and unpleasant. Recommendations by MAFF have been made to the shellfish industry suggesting cooking shellfish to a temperature of 85–90°C for 1½ mins. This kills Hepatitis A virus, and since 1988 there have been no major reports of viral illnesses from such heat-treated molluscs.

Oysters are eaten raw and cannot be subjected to heat treatment. Producers of oysters clean them by holding in tanks of clean water for forty-eight hours. While the oyster takes in water over its gills it is hoped that harmful organisms will be watered out. This will work for bacteria but not necessarily for virus, hence eating raw oysters remains a high risk.

Fruit and Vegetables: Using polluted water and sewage manure on fruit and vegetables for irrigation and fertilization is another potential source of primary viral contamination. Such soft fruits as raspberries have been identified in some outbreaks of Hepatitis A, as have some salad items.

Secondary Contamination

Food can be contaminated by infected food handlers. This is usually associated with cold food items that require the food handler to constantly handle them during preparation, e.g. sandwiches and salads.

DO buy shellfish, especially oysters from a reputable supplier.

DO keep them refrigerated until service.

HEPATITIS

Hepatitis means inflamed liver. There are four types of viral hepatitis, A, B, Non A/Non B and E. Of these only A is transmitted by food, E is a waterborne hepatitis.

Hepatitis A

This is a notifiable disease and accounts for 70% of all cases, but the proportion of cases caused by eating food is not known. The incubation period is long (3–6 weeks) so it is difficult to identify a food-borne source of infection unless the outbreak of food poisoning is clearly defined. The symptoms are fever, nausea, stomach pains and later jaundice. The duration of the illness can be anything from one week to several months and the severity of the symptoms varies. Fatalities are rare, and once infected the person is immune for life. The virus is spread by the faecal-oral route, so a food handler, who is a carrier of the disease and has poor hygiene standards, can contaminate the food.

Associating Hepatitis A with contaminated food is not always immediate and unfortunately with the limited technology available, it is not feasible to detect viruses in food, even if the food is suspect and subject to microbiological testing. Hepatitis E is a recently recognized form of hepatitis in underdeveloped countries where there have been some large-scale waterborne outbreaks with sewage-contaminated waters. There is some risk in shellfish imported from such countries.

INFECTIOUS DISEASES

The infectious diseases that we are concerned with are those that use food and water as vehicles for infections. They include bacteria, viruses, protozoa and parasitic worms. Food-borne infections usually fall into two main groups:

Usually Caught Abroad
Bacteria: typhoid, paratyphoid, cholera, brucellosis, tuberculosis, vibrio parahaemolyticus.
Protozoa: amoebic dysentery.
Worms: tapeworms, trichinosis

Newly Recognized Food-Borne Infections
Bacteria: campylobacter, listeria, yersinia, vtec.
Viruses: Hepatitis A.
Protozoa: giardia cryptosporidium.

ALLERGIES

Some people have allergies to certain foods but they will probably be aware of the problem as allergies usually start from an early age.

Common examples of foods that produce allergic reactions are dairy products and shellfish. The symptoms are usually sickness and diarrhoea.

Allergic reactions are not commonplace and are not the result of the food being poisoned.

5 Bacteria

INTRODUCTION

A micro-organism is a minute living thing, and can only be seen through a microscope. They include bacteria, viruses, rickettsia and protozoa. Bacteria can be seen with an ordinary optical microscope. Viruses are smaller than bacteria and can only be seen with a powerful electron microscope. They can only be grown on living cell tissue culture, live as parasites and can reproduce only in living cells of the plants or animals they infect. Rickettsia are life forms intermediate between bacteria and viruses, which cause typhus and other diseases. Protozoa are larger than bacteria.

The word germ is commonly used to describe any micro-organism that is capable of causing disease. Germs are also called pathogens or microbes. Pathogens are bacteria which are responsible for causing illness. Some pathogens cause food poisoning by growing and multiplying in food. Small numbers present in the food may be eaten without causing ill effects, but large numbers will invariably cause food poisoning.

Bacteria are tiny self-contained living organisms which can only be seen through a microscope. Approximately one million bacteria would cover a pinhead. Most bacteria are harmless and some are even helpful to man, but a small, very important proportion can infect some foods when conditions are suitable causing food poisoning and spoilage. Bacteria are present almost everywhere, in the air, on our skin and hair, in our food, kitchen equipment, in garden soil and in water. Some are mobile and can move in liquid but most cannot move by themselves and can only be transferred by direct contact.

Thousands of bacterial species are known. Many perform jobs vital to man such as degrading dead and waste materials, manufacturing cheese and yoghurt, fermenting certain foods and drinks, producing antibiotics, medicines and some vitamins in the human body. Only a few thousand types of bacteria are pathogenic and an even smaller number cause food poisoning.

Spoilage bacteria differ from food poisoning bacteria in that they are capable of spoiling food without making it poisonous. However conditions that allow food spoilage bacteria to grow and multiply, are also suitable for food poisoning bacteria. Spoilage bacteria are responsible for the change in the smell, taste and appearance of pasteurized milk when it goes 'off'. This is due to acids produced by the bacteria as they grow in the milk.

DO NOT use food that is obviously decaying. It may well just be spoilage bacteria, but don't take chances.

Bacteria that frequently cause food poisoning in Great Britain are salmonella, clostridium perfringens, staphylococcus aureus and bacillus cereus.

All bacteria have two names: the generic name (which comes first) and the specific name. The bacteria found in food are usually:

Spherical (cocci): A spherical or near spherical cell.
Bacillus: A rod-shaped cell longer than it is broad.
Vibrio: Curved rods shaped as 'commas'.

BACTERIAL GROWTH

Bacteria are living organisms and need food and water to survive in the same way that we do. There are four conditions that must be present if bacteria are to grow and multiply – food, moisture, warmth and time. Take any one of these factors away and bacterial growth slows down or stops. When these conditions are present the bacteria will grow and reproduce by splitting in two in a process called binary fission.

The bacterial cell grows by absorbing nutrients from its immediate environment and then splits to form two, new, identical cells. The bacteria will divide in two every twenty minutes, after six hours it is possible for one bacteria to become 262,144 and after twenty-four hours 7,000 million from the original one cell. The bacteria will continue to grow and multiply at the same rate until the food, or another essential condition, is no longer available.

BACILLUS

Any of a large group of rod-shaped bacteria. Many types of bacilli are harmless and are present in the air, water and soil, and within living organisms including human beings. Like all bacteria a bacillus is so small it can only be seen through a microscope. Most types of bacilli need oxygen to live and reproduce. Some become inactive for long periods of time in the form of spores, where conditions are unfavourable for growth.

A spore is a rounded body which forms inside the bacteria itself when conditions are unfavourable for growth (usually at high temperatures), e.g. boiling rice. The rest of the cell gradually disintegrates leaving the spore, as the food cools down from boiling point. This spore can resist very high temperatures and high concentration of chemicals that would kill any other bacteria; it can survive four hours at boiling point and is not destroyed by normal cooking methods. Spores will also form when other conditions are not favourable for growth, e.g. when there is no moisture present. Spores can survive for years with no food or moisture, then, when conditions are favourable again they will grow and multiply. Most bacteria are aerobes, needing air to survive. Some bacteria, including some that cause food poisoning, are anaerobes and can grow and multiply without air. Two types of food poisoning bacteria are anaerobes: clostridium perfringens and clostridium botulinum. Spore-forming bacteria and heat resistant, they are not killed off at high temperature.

Some of the diseases they cause are: bacillary dysentery, anthrax (a disease from cattle and sheep that can be transmitted to man), botulism, tuberculosis and typhoid fever. Many diseases caused by bacilli can be treated by antibiotics. Spore-forming bacteria are bacillus cereus, clostridium perfringens and clostridium botulinum.

DO be aware, when producing products that require boiling or stewing in a pan, that this cooking method drives out air. Stir the product frequently to ensure equal, thorough cooking of the food.

Bacteria are present on the skin, in the mouth and nose and some body passages (e.g. the bowels). Other bacteria, known as commensals, are harmless in these positions, however they can cause disease and food poisoning if they enter parts of the body where they are not usually found.

Incubation Period

The incubation period is the time that passes between the poisonous food entering the body and the onset of the first symptoms. The length of the incubation period helps to decide which type of bacteria has caused the food poisoning. The onset of these symptoms can be sudden, within two hours of the food being eaten, but there can be an interval of up to two days. The length of the incubation period also depends on the number of bacteria present. If the food is heavily contaminated, the incubation period will be shorter than if the food is contaminated with only half the number of the same type of bacteria.

Disease	Normal Incubation Period
Bacillary dysentery	7 days
Brucellosis	5–21 days
Hepatitis	15–50 days
Paratyphoid	1–10 days
Salmonellosis	5–48 hours
Trichomoniasis	4–20 days
Typhoid	7–20 days

SALMONELLA

Between the years 1909–23 many of the bacteria now known to be responsible for most of our food poisoning outbreaks were grouped together under the name salmonella, in honour of the American vet Dr Salmon who discovered the first member of the group in 1885. More outbreaks of food poisoning are caused by salmonella than any other bacteria, over 25,000 were reported in 1989. The symptoms can be severe and cause approximately fifty deaths each year. The high-risk groups are most at risk of dying should they suffer salmonella food poisoning.

Salmonella causes infective food poisoning and large numbers must be present in the food when it is eaten. The bacteria pass into the digestive system, some are destroyed by the acids in the stomach but others are protected by the food and pass into the small intestine where they will multiply. As the numbers increase some bacteria die and produce a toxin, which causes diarrhoea, vomiting and fever accompanied by headaches. In 1–2% of reported cases a more generalized infection occurs. Because of the length of time the bacteria take to increase to a level which causes the symptoms, the incubation period is usually twelve to seventy-two hours. The symptoms in most people last from one to ten days but some people can be ill for much longer, and even after recovery the victim can carry the salmonella bacteria in their faeces for long periods.

Salmonella is commonly found in animal fodder and in the intestines of many animals including cattle, pigs and poultry. Mice, rats, pets, flies and birds carry salmonella in their intestines and on their fur and feet.

Salmonella is brought into the kitchen in raw foods, particularly raw meat and poultry, unpasteurized milk and eggs. Other raw foods, including vegetables and spices, have occasionally been found to be contaminated. The food handler can sometimes be an unknowing carrier of salmonella and thus contaminate food if they do not wash their hands after visiting the toilet. The bacteria will be present in their intestines and faeces. Salmonella is not a spore-forming bacteria and it is readily killed by heat at temperatures above 65°C.

A common cause of salmonella food poisoning is inadequate thawing of frozen poultry. If any ice is present in the centre of the chicken it is not defrosted and a great deal of heat energy is used to melt the ice. It takes longer then for the internal temperature to equal the external temperature of the chicken, so by the end of the cooking time the temperature of the inside of the bird is not high enough to kill the bacteria and the warm temperature encourages growth.

Example of salmonella outbreak:

Seventy clients and staff at a day centre were taken ill twenty-four hours after eating vol-au-vents. One person died and eight were admitted to hospital. Frozen chickens weighing 3–3½ lb were not defrosted thoroughly. They were left overnight at room temperature covered in foil, then roasted for 1–1½ hours at gas mark 6–7, then the temperature was lowered to gas mark 3 for 2 hours. They were left to cook for 1½ hours on the top of the oven, then moved near an open window for 19 hours. The next day the chickens were cut up and minced to make the vol-au-vent filling; these were then reheated at 55°C before they were served.

Inadequate defrosting and cooking combined with rewarming and a long cooling period at room temperature can produce salmonella. In this case high levels of bacteria in the vol-au-vents of 10 million per gm were recorded.

DO thaw frozen poultry and joints of meat thoroughly before cooking.
DO cook food thoroughly for a long enough time and at a high enough temperature.

STAPHYLOCOCCUS AUREAS

This bacteria causes toxic food poisoning and is not a spore-forming bacteria. At 'danger zone' temperatures the bacteria will grow and multiply and produce a toxin. When the food is eaten the toxin will irritate the stomach lining, causing severe vomiting, sometimes followed by collapse.

The onset of illness is rapid, usually within 1–7 hours, more often 2–6 hours. The illness is rarely fatal, and the illness is now less common that it used to be.

The toxin is more heat resistant than the bacteria itself. Whereas the bacteria is readily killed by heat (1–2 minutes boiling), the toxin can withstand up to 30 minutes in boiling water. Lightly cooked food may therefore contain active toxins.

Staphylococcus aureas is found in the nose, throat and on the skin of 50% of the population, and also found in septic cuts, spots and boils on the skin. Food handlers carrying the bacteria will bring the bacteria into the kitchen by directly touching food, sneezing and coughing over food, through cuts not covered by a waterproof dressing, touching septic spots and then touching food, and by fingers infected by 'picking the nose' then touching food.

The food handler is usually the person responsible for contaminating the food with staphylococcus aureas and the foods affected are those that have been cooked and are then eaten cold or only given minimal heating, e.g. cold meats and cream dishes (trifles, custards and other milk products). Staphylococcus aureas has the ability to grow in high concentrations of salt, which is unusual for bacteria, so outbreaks involving salty foods like ham are often caused by staphylococcus aureas.

An example:

A ham was cooked in the evening and then transferred to an open press and left. The next day it was placed in a refrigerator. That evening the ham was used to make sandwiches. Eleven men were taken ill three hours after eating the sandwiches; five were admitted to hospital. On investigation it was discovered that the food handler had a heavy cold and staphylococcus aureas bacteria were isolated from a nasal swab.

DO NOT allow food handlers to handle food excessively.
DO use tongs for food that will not be heated again.
DO NOT leave meat sandwiches at room temperature. Refrigerate them.
DO insist on high standards of food hygiene.
DO NOT allow food handlers to touch their nose, mouth or hair.

TYPHOID

Typhoid fever is caused by the bacteria salmonella typhi. It causes a more severe type of illness than the food poisoning caused by the majority of species of the salmonella group. Unlike any other salmonellae, man is the natural source of these bacteria and the infection is passed on in the human faeces or sewage. Typhoid fever is rare in Great Britain but occasionally people suffer from it on returning from abroad.

The incubation period is 7–21 days and the symptoms are characterised by a high fever lasting 2–3 weeks or more. There are rose-coloured spots on the body and severe diarrhoea which usually starts in the second or third week of the fever. Death may result if not treated, although this is rare in Britain. In most people after recovering from typhoid fever, the body is totally free from the bacteria that caused the illness, but in a few people the bacteria persists, usually in the gall bladder and occasionally in the bone marrow. These 'stores' release typhoid bacteria into the intestines or the blood stream, and are excreted in the faeces or urine. A carrier can contaminate food by the faecal-oral route or infected urine may get into drinking water.

An example:

A typhoid epidemic near London in 1938 was caused by contamination of a reservoir where the sterilizing plant was temporarily out of action.

Between 200–300 cases of typhoid and paratyphoid are reported each year in Great Britain, most of the patients reported catching the disease from abroad or from someone close to them who had been abroad.

There have been instances of shellfish and watercress grown in sewage-contaminated water causing typhoid fever, but regulations concerning shellfish have almost eliminated them as a cause of typhoid fever.

DO wash all vegetables thoroughly, particularly watercress which may have been grown in sewage-contaminated water.

PARATYPHOID

Paratyphoid fever is caused by the bacteria salmonella paratyphi. It causes a more severe type of illness than the food poisoning caused by the majority of the species of the genus salmonellae.

Salmonella paratyphi is a parasite of man only, unlike other salmonellae which are only found in animals; if an outbreak occurs we know that a human carrier must be involved. Paratyphoid fever is similar to typhoid fever but the symptoms are generally less severe. The incubation period is one to ten days and the symptoms are fever and diarrhoea. The disease can be caused by food handlers who are carriers of the bacteria, via the faecal-oral route; drinking water that is contaminated by, or has been contaminated by, sewage; or food gathered from contaminated water.

In January 1988 there was an outbreak of paratyphoid fever in England that was traced to an Indian Independence Day celebration in Birmingham. It was attended by more than 1,000 people. Environmental Health Officers became aware of the problem when people started to become ill. Eleven victims were hospitalized, some of whom were seriously ill, and they managed to trace five hundred guests at the party. They then issued a nationwide alert to trace the remainder. They asked for anyone suffering from fever, diarrhoea, headaches or generally feeling unwell to contact them. The food on the menu was lamb curry, Indian sweetmeats, mixed vegetables and rice. The EHOs found that the food had been prepared in totally unsuitable premises and under totally unsuitable conditions. The food had been prepared the day before the party and left overnight for fifteen to sixteen hours, in a factory with no proper washing facilities and whose conditions were ideal for the bacteria to grow and multiply.

LISTERIA (Lysteria Monocytogenes)

Outbreaks of listeriosis are becoming more common and the World Health Organization now believes that contaminated food is a major source of the organism. It is believed that the true annual figure is 500–600 cases of listeria each year in England and Wales. For the first time since convenience foods were invented, it has been realized that they are as convenient to bacteria as they are to people. For many years cases were thought to result from contact with infected animals, in spite of the fact that most patients gave no history of such contact. Listeria is found everywhere in the environment, it is found in cultivated and uncultivated soils, vegetation and silage (Scottish researchers found they could culture it from garden grass quite easily and if farmers make silage badly, listeria thrives), surface water and raw untreated sewage. An increasing problem in sheep, if their manure is used carelessly listeria can be found in vegetables.

Listeria will survive on the ground for several months in sewage sludge. It is found in rivers and streams, and water used for the irrigation of salad and other crops may spread the bacteria. It is fairly common in milk, but pasteurization kills it. It should not be present in hazardous levels in fresh salad but you are advised to wash all vegetables well before use.

The bacteria has also been found in many species of wild and domestic animals, birds, fish, crustaceans and insects. Listeria in human faeces of the general population may reach 5%, but rates can be considerably higher in the faeces of veterinary, abbatoir and certain laboratory workers. Most cases of listeriosis in humans have been associated with persons who are already suffering with impaired immunity, e.g. cancer, transplant and AIDS patients. They are usually treated at first for meningitis and/or septicaemia, but the disease is becoming more frequent in apparently healthy individuals although to succumb to the disease one must have received a mass onslaught of the bacteria. The infection of women who are pregnant presents a 'flu-like' illness which may lead to spontaneous abortion, stillbirth or premature delivery and neonatal sepsis. Despite the availability of effective antibiotics, overall mortality rates following infection are 30%. Listeria can survive and multiply at refrigeration temperatures (4°C). Convenience-chilled foods, longer shelf lives and greater availability means that the potential exists for the bacteria to reach high levels in certain products. There is evidence that listeria is more virulent when grown at refrigeration temperatures. Food manufacturers have responded to public demand for less additives in food and have returned to the more traditional methods of preserving foods such as high salt content or acidity. Listeria not only survives but grows at high salt concentration and pH5.

There is much controversy surrounding establishing a 'safe threshold' for listeria in food. The World Health Organization believes there should be no listeria in 25 gms of food. Unfortunately, microbiological sampling of the food (usually performed shortly after production) with present culture techniques generally does not detect levels in listeria at below 100 organisms per gm. So if we assume 1-3 days in production and a mean doubling time of 12–24 hours, a refrigerated product containing 10 organisms per gm after 10 days can have 10 to the power of 6 organisms per gm. Cook chill producers have DHSS 1981 guidelines to follow. Their products are available in all major supermarket outlets, and many of these products and their storage conditions contravene these guidelines. Certain recommendations (by Professor Richard Lacey and Dr Kevin Kerr from the Department of Microbiology at the University of Leeds) have now been put forward:

Listeriosis should be made a notifiable disease;
Cook chill products should not be kept under refrigeration temperature for more than three days;
Retail outlets should comply with Department of Health guidelines concerning refrigerated storage, and should remove from sale and destroy all products being held at 4°C. Temperature control should be measured by probing the food itself;
Current DOH guidelines should be amended to include listeria monocytogenes in microbiological monitoring of cook chill products;
The duration and end point temperature of the current methods of heating (or reheating) food stuffs should show all listeria is destroyed;
Cook chill catering should be suspended in hospitals, until the safety of this method is proved.

Until these recommendations are implemented any refrigerated foods found to contain listeria in 25 gms should be declared 'unfit for human consumption'.

In July 1992 more than twenty people died and ninety-nine became seriously ill in an outbreak of listeria food poisoning in France. A French spokesman said that 'the cause is almost certain to be a mass branded product, probably a cheese or prepared dish like pâté, with a national distribution, which would account for the wide episodic spread of the outbreak.' French authorities had difficulty detecting the source of the outbreak since symptoms may not appear for six weeks, by which time the contaminated food would usually have been thrown away. Official French figures have not been updated since June 1992 and unconfirmed reports say they are as high as thirty-four dead, which would make it the second most serious (confirmed) outbreak of listeria food poisoning.

DO NOT use unpasteurized milk and cream. When bottles or containers have been opened, protect from dust.
DO keep cheeses covered to prevent cross contamination.
DO ensure pregnant women, the high-risk groups and those with impaired immunity avoid eating soft cheeses and meat pâté.
DO ensure all fresh chickens are cooked thoroughly.
DO check 'use by' dates on chilled food.
DO NOT allow the storage temperature to rise above 3°C for chilled products.
DO NOT store for more than two days before use.
DO wash all fruit, vegetables and salads before use and *always* ensure all food handlers maintain high standards of personal hygiene while involved in handling food.

DYSENTERY

There are two types of dysentery, amoebic and bacillary. Amoebic dysentery is rare in Europe, but endemic in some tropical countries, especially where sanitation and hygiene are poor. This dysentery is spread by the faecal-oral route or from contaminated water or food. Bacilliary dysentery is caused by a bacteria from the shigella group and is responsible for a large number of outbreaks in Great Britain. Shigella lives only in man, so when an outbreak occurs, it is established at once that a human carrier is involved.

The incubation period is one to seven days and the symptoms are watery diarrhoea and fever. The disease is caused by personal contact and the faecal-oral route. Bacterial dysentery can spread very quickly in schools and institutions if hand-washing facilities are poor or inadequate, or personal hygiene standards are low. Persons who are carriers of shigella and do not wash their hands after visiting the toilet will transmit the bacteria.

In May 1992 it was reported there was an outbreak of dysentery in the north of England. Some 6,000 cases were reported, the majority of which were preschool and school children. Children may forget to wash their hands properly after visiting the toilet or the hand-washing facilities may be inadequate in play groups, toddler groups or schools. Children will put their hands in their mouths (or another child's mouth!) and transmit the bacteria to another. One school of thought on this outbreak is 'that with the advent of soft toilet tissue, a child with the onset of dysentery will have quite watery diarrhoea, and after using this type of toilet paper, which is also porous, the child will have hundreds of thousands of the bacteria on his hands and even quite thorough hand washing will not remove all the bacteria and so will transmit the bacteria.'

DO ensure the staff fill in a health review questionnaire after returning from a holiday abroad.
DO ensure you provide sufficient hand-washing facilities for staff and customers.
DO (if you deal with children) teach thorough washing of the hands.

E.COLI

E.Coli (Eschericia Coli 0157) is a rod-shaped bacteria. It is always present in the intestinal tract of healthy people and is not normally pathogenic, but there are some sero-types of vero-cytoxin producing E.Coli, and entro-toxigenic forms of the bacteria (E.Tech), which produce a heat-stable toxin in the intestine. In recent years human illness from E.Coli has been showing a steady increase in Great Britain and a similar rising trend has been noticed in North America.

E. Coli 0157 is by far the most common sero group in human infections and was first described in Canada in 1977. Their association with human disease was confirmed in 1982–3. Vero-cytoxin producing E.Coli have also been implicated as a cause of disease in animals, particularly calves and pigs, but the 0157 strains do not appear to cause significant illness in animals.

E.Coli is used extensively in laboratories as an indicator organism in food analysis. The presence of E.Coli in food indicates the food has been contaminated by a faecal source and is therefore a risk to humans. The symptoms of E.Coli food poisoning range from mild diarrhoea to a severe bloody diarrhoea (haemorrahagic colitis) and a proportion of patients will go on to develop haemolytic uraemic syndrome – acute kidney failure. All age groups are affected but it is most common in young children (under two years old). The illness lasts from one to five days. The bacteria is heat sensitive and is readily killed by thorough cooking.

In 1991 a highly significant link was made between an outbreak of E.Coli food poisoning in the Preston area with beefburgers. Seven sufferers had eaten beefburgers at a particular catering outlet before becoming ill.

Whereas E.Coli food poisoning is still quite rare, there were 300 cases in 1990 in Great Britain, and the rising trend in North America is linked with eating beefburgers.

DO cook all beefburgers/hamburgers thoroughly and any other similar minced beef products. Homemade beefburgers should be cooked until the juices run clear and there are no pink bits inside.

DO, if buying beefburgers in packs, follow the manufacturer's instructions on cooking. If buying from a butcher, cook them thoroughly. There is no need for further precautions so long as these meat products are thoroughly cooked.

CHOLERA

This is an acute epidemic disease caused by a bacteria and spread by the faecal-oral route. Cholera is caught by drinking polluted water or eating contaminated food. It occurs mainly in countries that lack modern sanitary techniques, such as frequent testing and purification of water supplies and proper sewage disposal.

The bacteria responsible is vibrio cholerae. The symptoms are the sudden onset of very severe diarrhoea and vomiting; the diarrhoea is sometimes referred to as ricewater stools. The resulting dehydration is often fatal. Treatment consists of combating the dehydration with large quantities of a special salt solution directly into the vein. Where medical facilities are poor, patients can be treated by directly drinking this solution. All visitors to countries where cholera is common should be vaccinated against the disease, but it is only effective for a few months and requires revaccination every six months. If you or your staff visit a country where cholera occurs:

DO use only boiled or bottled water.
DO check food is not contaminated by flies or hands.
DO NOT eat uncooked fruit and vegetables.
DO NOT add ice cubes to drinks.
DO fill in a review health questionnaire for all staff returning from holidays abroad.

CLOSTRIDIUM PERFRINGENS

There are approximately 1,000 cases of clostridium perfringens (previously known as clostridium welchi) reported each year making it the second most common form of food poisoning. It is a spore-forming, anaerobic bacteria. It does not produce toxins when multiplying in the danger zone, but when it is eaten spores are formed and a toxin which irritates the intestinal wall is released, causing diarrhoea. This is not the same as toxic food poisoning or infective food poisoning but has some characteristics of both.

The incubation period is longer than with toxic food

poisoning (as in staphylococcus aureas) and shorter than infective food poisoning (as in salmonella). The incubation period is from 8 to 22 hours (usually 12–18) and when the bacteria reach the intestines they form a spore and release a toxin. The symptoms are abdominal pain and diarrhoea; the patient rarely vomits and the symptoms and the duration of the illness last 12–24 hours. Clostridium perfringens can often be found in the intestines of animals (including humans) and spores can be found in the soil.

Flies and bluebottles are usually heavily infected with clostridium perfringens. It enters the kitchen on raw meat and raw vegetables, particularly when coated with soil. Clostridium perfringens brought into the kitchen in this way can be transferred to cooked food by careless food handling. The meat itself may cause food poisoning as clostridium perfringens can survive the cooking process. Vegetables coated with soil or dust from sacking or packing cases may contaminate other foods. Food handlers may be carrying clostridium perfringens in their intestines and spread the bacteria into food if hands are not washed after visiting the toilet.

The spores of clostridium perfringens are not destroyed by normal cooking methods; they can survive boiling, steaming, stewing or braising for up to four hours. The spores are not then multiplying, but if the food is cooled slowly or kept in danger zone temperatures they can divide in two every twelve minutes. The spores will germinate producing vegetative bacteria which will multiply rapidly, but there is little growth below °10C.

As this bacteria is an anaerobe, it is frequently found reproducing rapidly at the bottom of a luke-warm stew or stock-pot, or large food masses where there is little air, e.g. large meat joints, meat pies, minced meat dishes. Reheated meat dishes are also a frequent cause of clostridium perfringens food poisoning, since the spore it forms will survive each reheating process.

In a factory canteen food handlers are preparing lunch for the shift workers. The first shift will eat at 11.00 a.m., the second at 2.00 p.m. One of the dishes on the menu is beef stew. The stew was prepared by a chef using beef, onions, carrots and swedes. He cuts up all the ingredients and puts them in a large pan to simmer. He regularly turns the pan and the stew cooks for 3 hours 30 minutes. Before the end of the cooking time mushrooms were added. The first shift ate at 11.00 a.m. but not all the stew was eaten. It was put in heated containers to store for the 2.00 p.m. shift. That night thirty people were taken ill with severe stomach pains and diarrhoea. An outbreak of food poisoning was confirmed caused by clostridium perfringens and traced to the stew. Only people on the 2.00 p.m. shift were affected. The reasons for this outbreak were that the centre of the stew was not properly heated, allowing the spores to germinate and the bacteria to multiply. It was then stored in danger zone conditions.

DO handle meat away from other foods to avoid cross contamination.
DO cover food to prevent dust and insects contaminating it.
DO prepare potatoes and root vegetables away from other foods to avoid cross contamination from the soil on them.
DO prepare meat dishes on the day they are to be eaten and serve hot. If this is not possible, cool the food quickly and refrigerate. Reheat thoroughly until piping hot.
DO NOT add hot gravy to cold meat.
DO NOT attempt to cook joints of meat over 3 kg in weight to ensure thorough heat penetration.

CLOSTRIDIUM BOTULINUM

In addition to those conditions already described in clostridium perfringens, there is a food poisoning caused by clostridium botulinum which fortunately is rare, but very serious and greatly feared, because 70% of all cases are fatal. Surviving cases take months to recover. The victim's life can be saved by administering antitoxin very soon after the onset of the illness. The bacteria is very similar in appearance to clostridium perfringens. It is a rod-shaped bacteria, anaerobic and forms a spore where conditions are unfavourable for growth. Therefore faulty canned, bottled or vacuum-packed foods are at a special risk. Any food product with evidence of gas inside, like blown cans, should be discarded immediately. Most cases of botulism have occured after eating understerilized canned food, or food in faulty cans that have been contaminated after sterilization. Understerilization leads to the bacteria multiplying producing a gas in the can leading to the characteristic bulging of the can. It is quite rare for commercially canned foods to contain this bacteria, but in the USA home canning is still practised and there have been cases of food poisoning from canned vegetables.

The toxin the spores produce is highly poisonous and people have died after eating only a mouthful of the infected food. The incubation period is 24–72 hours and death follows within 1–8 days unless the patient is given an antitoxin soon after the symptoms appear. Recovery from the illness is slow, from 6 to 8 months. The symptoms of clostridiumn botulinum are giddiness, double vision and headaches. Diarrhoea may be present at first but later the patient is constipated, the central nervous system is affected after the bacteria enter the blood stream, and the throat muscles contract and become paralysed, making talking difficult. Death is usually from respiratory failure.

Clostridium botulinum lives in the soil, but it is not found in the intestines of animals. It has been found in fish, particularly from the waters around Japan where fermented fish is a delicacy. Although clostridium botulinum produces a spore, it is not heat resistant and the toxin it produces is readily killed by boiling it for a few minutes.

There is no danger these days from commercially canned products so long as damaged or blown cans are rejected. In the past most cases of botulism occured after eating understerilized canned food which was subsequently not reheated sufficiently to destroy the toxin.

There have been twenty outbreaks of clostridium botulinum this century, with six outbreaks in the past twenty years. A recent outbreak occured in and around the Lancashire area. The outbreak was traced to a yoghurt manufacturer using contaminated hazelnut purée. The hazelnuts were imported from Turkey, Spain and Portugal, and then made into a purée in a fruit-processing plant in Kent, before being transported in sealed containers to the yoghurt manufacturers. Ten people including four children became seriously ill after eating the hazelnut yoghurt, and it was confirmed as the worst outbreak of clostridium botulinum for more than sixty years. All the victims were hospitalized; three victims, a girl aged three, a boy of thirteen and an adult aged twenty, were supported on ventilation machines.

The outbreak previous to the Lancashire case involved a man from the south of England who became ill after eating a meal on an aeroplane. The man aged fifty contracted clostridium botulinum after eating a kosher meal on a flight in 1987. The meal included rice and vegetables. He became totally paralysed and was put on a life-support machine; his muscles, eyesight and hearing were affected and he was unable to talk. He spent seven months in hospital and a further month in a rehabilitation centre learning to stand up and walk again. It took him a year to recover sufficiently to enable him to go back to work at his sedentary job. He still attends a gym three times a week to build up his muscles and reflexes. He was suing the airline.

Two pensioners from Birmingham died in 1978 after eating tinned red salmon and two others were made seriously ill. The company involved in the manufacture of the red salmon paid out undisclosed compensation in an out-of-court settlement. The slump in the sales of this company's red salmon cost them £2 million.

The worst outbreak in Great Britain was in 1922 at Lochmaree in the Scottish Highlands. Six fishermen died after eating sandwiches containing contaminated duck paste.

Other foods implicated in outbreaks of botulism have included macaroni cheese and pickled fish.

DO NOT use canned foods which show any signs of bulging or have seams which are leaking or discoloured, have denting or rusting.
DO reject any blown cans.
DO NOT attempt to can your own produce.
DO NOT refreeze defrosting frozen vegetables. Cook frozen vegetables from frozen.
DO keep smoked fish frozen.
DO keep vacuum packed meats, fish and vegetables refrigerated or frozen before use.

BACILLUS CEREUS

This is an aerobic bacteria which grows only in the presence of air and is a heat-resistant, spore-forming bacteria. It is frequently found in dried foods such as cereals and rice. As an aerobe the bacteria will not grow and multiply in the dried foods but will remain dormant. When the food is being cooked the bacteria protects itself from the high temperatures by forming a spore to survive the cooking process. If the food is then left to cool down and left in 'danger zone' temperatures the spores are released. The bacteria grow and multiply, produce a toxin which quickly spreads through the food, this toxin irritates the stomach lining, causing vomiting; the attack can occur very suddenly, within 1–2 hours of the food being eaten, but it is over very quickly.

Another type of bacillus cereus food poisoning is quite rare in Great Britain. This causes diarrhoeal symptoms and is produced in the intestines, but the amount of toxins produced depends on the number of bacteria eaten, it is destroyed by heat and probably cannot survive the acids produced by the stomach.

The toxin-producing, vomiting form of bacillus cereus is very heat resistent and is produced in the food. It can survive pressure cooking for 1½ hours and frying for short periods.

DO cool cooked foods quickly then refrigerate or keep them hot for service above 63°C.
DO cook rice in small batches, keep it hot and serve as soon as possible.
DO when reheating meat or rice dishes, reheat until piping hot, above 70°C and serve immediately.
DO NOT batch cook rice and leave it in 'danger zone' temperatures, refrigerate.
DO NOT reheat meat or rice dishes more than once – throw it away!

CAMPYLOBACTER

During the 1970s the development of new laboratory techniques allowed detailed examination of this group of bacteria. These bacteria were identified as a seperate family and given the name campylobacter derived from the Greek *kampulos*, meaning curved, and *bakterion*, meaning rod. The campylobacter jejuni are slim rods, either spiral- or S-shaped and can move rapidly through fluids. It grows best under reduced oxygen conditions.

The first report of campylobacter jejuni in England and Wales was in 1977 and was identified as the cause of a human gastroenteritis and is now believed to be the most common cause of intestinal infection in the UK today. Since the 1980s reported cases of campylobacter jejuni have exceeded those of salmonella. In 1988 there were 29,000 reported cases in England and Wales. The illness, although unpleasant, is comparatively mild and has caused very few deaths.

The symptoms may start suddenly with abdominal pains, followed by smelly, sometimes blood-stained, diarrhoea; fever, headaches and dizziness are also common. The diarrhoea can last up to three days and the other symptoms for several days more. The infective dose is small so the organism does not need to multiply to any great numbers to cause illness.

The bacteria are smaller than other bacteria found in the intestines of humans, and have been found in cattle, pigs, poultry and domestic pets. It is rarely spread from adult to adult but it may be passed from child to parent or parent to child. Human infection has been linked to drinking contaminated water, unpasteurized milk, contact with cats and dogs with diarrhoea, eating undercooked chicken, and campylobacter jejuni has even been isolated from coastal sea water.

DO ensure high standards of personal and food hygiene.
DO cook food thoroughly; this bacteria is easily killed by heat.
DO defrost frozen poultry completely and do use pasteurized milk.

YERSINIA ENTEROCOLYTICA

Yersinia is now thought to be more common in the UK than recent reporting suggests and is frequently reported as the cause of diarrhoea in some Scandinavian and European countries. It is a rod-shaped bacteria, which like listeria can grow slowly at refrigeration temperatures.

The main symptom which occurs 24–36 hours after eating the contaminated food is diarrhoea. Other symptoms can include severe abdominal pain, sometimes mistaken for appendicitis, fever and vomiting. Many animals carry yersinia in their digestive tract, and this bacteria has been found in milk and dairy products, meats (particularly pork) and vegetables.

DO ensure thorough cooking of all meat products.
DO store relevant foods at temperatures below 4°C.

6 Legislation

SUMMARY OF ACTS

There are now two Acts in force which have given Local Authorities' Environmental Health Officers new enforcing powers. They concern all caterers from hot-dog salesmen and corner shops to multinational hotels and restaurants. The two Acts are the Food Safety Act 1990 and the Food Hygiene (Amendment) Regulations 1989.

The law says: 'It is an offence to sell or possess for sale, food which is not of a nature, quality or substance demanded by the customer, and/or which fails to comply with the legal requirements and/or which is likely to cause food poisoning'. You can be fined up to £20,000 for each serious offence.

The Food Hygiene Regulations control the standards of hygiene in premises and are divided into these sections:

Premises
'Your premises must be kept clean, pest-proof and in good repair, they should have adequate lighting.'

Equipment
'Must not be made of an absorbent material such as wood, they must be kept clean and in good condition.'

Food Handlers
'Must keep themselves clean, cover cuts and sores with a waterproof dressing, wear suitable clothing, must not smoke or spit, and must report any illness to their employers.'

DO insist on your staff wearing clean clothing to work.
DO provide waterproof dressings of a distinctive colour.
DO insist on suitable, appropriate overclothing for your business.

DO set up a reporting procedure for staff to ring in, when they suspect they are suffering the symptoms of food poisoning or septic cuts or boils.
DO NOT allow smoking, spitting or chewing in the food handling area.

Services
'Businesses must supply first-aid materials, somewhere to keep outdoor clothing, a satisfactory supply of hot and cold water. Toilets must be well lit, clean and ventilated. A washhand basin with soap, nail-brush and drying facilities must be provided situated between the toilet and the food area.'

DO check your first-aid box for contents. See p. 174.

Methods
'High-risk foods must be kept outside the danger zone, all open foods offered for sale must be kept covered, avoid exposing foods to the risk of cross contamination.'

Penalties
A fine of up to £20,000 for each serious breach of the Food Safety Act; for more serious offences up to two years in prison plus unlimited fines. You can be forced to comply by an improvement order or an emergency prohibition order which involves closing all or part of the business.

Due Diligence
The Food Safety Act allows the defence of 'due diligence', provided you have taken all reasonable precautions, such as setting up a system to ensure checks are being made with which you and your staff try to comply. Provided problems are noted and action taken, you have exercised 'due diligence'.

COSHH

Under the Control of Substances Hazardous to Health Regulations 1988 (COSHH) employers must:

Assess the risk to the health of their workers from any

substances they handle in the course of their work. This means that the employer, or someone they appoint, must know the product handled by their employees and know if any of the products propose a hazard.

Introduce measures to prevent or control the risk of handling hazardous chemicals. This may be achieved by changing a hazardous preparation to one with minimal risk by providing protective clothing or equipment to reduce the risk.

Inform employees of the risk of hazardous substances. This warning may be in the form of a memo, which must be read and signed, or a notice in the workplace where the product is used.

Train employees to work safely. New employees must be shown how to use the products and supervised until they can use them safely.

Ensure hazardous chemicals are used and stored safely; they should be stored in clearly marked cupboards or storerooms. If transferred to smaller containers, ensure that the smaller containers are clearly labelled with the contents and correct usage.

The law covering food hygiene in all food premises is contained in the regulations covered by the *Food Hygiene (General) Regulations 1970,* with amendments made by the *Food Hygiene (Amendment) Regulations 1990* and the *Food Safety Act 1990.*

The Food Hygiene (Amendment) Regulations came into force on 1 April 1991 and The Food Safety Act 1990 came into force on 1 January 1991 and made substantial changes to strengthen and update the previous regulations. The new Act has a number of enabling powers that allow a minister to make further regulations and issue Codes of Practice.

A breach of any of the following regulations will result in the issue of an Improvement Order (Section 10), a Prohibition Order (Section 11) and/or prosecution.

The main requirements of the Regulations relate to the cleanliness of premises and equipment; hygienic food handling practices; personal hygiene of food handlers; construction, repair and maintenance of premises; water supply and washing facilities; water disposal; and temperature control of certain foods.

All references to 'regulations' are covered by the Food Hygiene (General) Regulations 1970.

All references to 'section' are covered by the Food Safety Act 1990.

FOOD SAFETY ACT 1990

Part 1 Preliminary

SECTION 1

FOOD: THE MEANING OF FOOD AND OTHER BASIC EXPRESSIONS

Food has a very wide definition under the Act. It includes anything that is eaten, drunk or sold as a food product. It excludes:

Live animals or birds;
Live fish (unless normally eaten alive e.g. elvers);
Fodder or feeding stuffs for animals, birds or fish;
Medicines.

The definition of food also covers tap water and foods of no nutritional value which are eaten including:

Releasing agents used in bakeries to help remove baked bread from tins;
Food colourings and food additives;
Bulking agents, used as ingredients in some processed foods;
Chewing gum.

Slimming aids, vitamin supplements and herbal remedies are all also defined as food.

FOOD PREMISES

Food premises mean any premises used for the purpose of a food business.

Food business includes the undertaking of a canteen, club, school, hospital or institution, whether carried on for profit or not, and any undertaking or activity carried on by a local or public authority.

Commercial operation means any of thc following:

Selling, possessing for sale, and offering, exposing or advertising for sale;

Consigning, delivering or serving by way of sale;
Preparing for sale or presenting, labelling or wrapping for the purpose of sale;
Storing or transporting for the purpose of sale;
Importing and exporting.
Premises also include any place, any vehicle, stall or movable structure.

SECTION 2

FOOD SALES: *EXTENDED MEANING OF SALE:*
Under the Food Safety Act this section applies to any food supplied by the food business. This is taken to be a sale of food.

The Act also applies to any food offered as a prize, reward or given away as part of any entertainment to which the public are admitted, whether payment of money is received or not; and to food offered for advertising purposes for any trade or business, as a prize or reward, or given away whether money is received or not. It also applies to any food deposited or exposed in any premises with the purpose of being offered or given away or that has been exposed for sale by the occupier of the premises.
Entertainment includes any social gathering, amusement, exhibition, performance, game, sport, or trial of skill.

SECTION 3

FOOD INTENDED FOR HUMAN CONSUMPTION
Food intended for human consumption should be fit to eat. Unfit food includes mouldy food, decomposing food and food containing food poisoning organisms or excessive additives. Contaminated food includes that containing foreign bodies, insects or rodent droppings.

SECTION 4

Defines various ministers having duties, functions, powers and responsibilities under the Act.

SECTION 5

DEFINES THE ENFORCEMENT AUTHORITIES AND AUTHORIZED OFFICERS

Authorized officers of local authorities enforce the law relating to food safety. They have certain powers to achieve improved food safety. The authorized officer is most likely to be an Environmental Health Officer, but it can be another officer of the local authority with experience and technical ability relating to food safety and hygiene. All officers have to be authorized in writing and will carry some form of identification, which will state the legislation under which they have the power to act.

They have the right to enter premises at all reasonable hours and to examine records or equipment.

They have the power to issue improvement notices and emergency prohibition notices.

They can recommend legal proceedings are taken.

They have the right to inspect, detain or seize food suspected of not complying with Food Safety regulations.

They must have regard to the Codes of Practice drawn up in relation to each of these aspects of an officer's powers.

SECTION 6

Enforcement of the Act.
See Codes of Practice No. 1.

Part 2 Provisions
Food Safety

SECTION 7

RENDERING FOOD INJURIOUS TO HEALTH: FOOD SAFETY OFFENCES

There are two groups:

1 Rendering food injurious to health is an offence by any of the following:

Adding any substance to food or using any ingredients in the

preparation of food which would make it harmful to health, e.g. adding ethylene glycol (antifreeze) to wine to improve its sweetness;
Taking away any constituent from food making it harmful to health;
Processing food or treating it to make it harmful, with intent to sell the food for human consumption, e.g. improper irradiation, or using insecticide to fumigate infested food.
The definition of harmful to health will include any impairment whether permanent or temporary.

2 Selling food not complying with food safety requirements. Food fails to comply if:
It has been rendered harmful to health (as in Section 7, Part 1);
It is unfit for human consumption;
It is so contaminated that it would not be expected to be used for human consumption.
It is an offence to sell, offer, display, advertise or even possess food which does not comply with the above.

SECTION 8

SELLING FOOD NOT COMPLYING WITH FOOD SAFETY REQUIREMENTS
Any person who sells, offers, exposes, advertises or has in his possession food intended for sale or for preparation for such sale, or deposits or consigns to another person for sale, which fails to comply with the requirements shall be guilty of an offence.
Food fails to comply if:
It has been rendered injurious to health;
It is unfit for human consumption;
It is so contaminated that it would not be reasonable to expect it to be used for human consumption in that state.
If the food is part of a batch, lot or consignment and fails to comply, it will be presumed that all of that food will fail to comply. This will include any part of a product derived from an animal which has been slaughtered in a knackers' yard; or if the carcass has been brought into the yard.

SECTION 9

Inspection and seizure of food: An authorized officer may at all times inspect any food intended for human consumption. If on inspection he decides the food fails to comply with food safety regulations he can either:
Give notice that the food is not to be used or removed except to a place specified in the notice.
Seize the food and remove it to be dealt with by a Justice of the Peace.

If the officer exercises these powers, he should within twenty-one days decide whether or not the food complies. If he is satisfied he should withdraw the notice; if not satisfied he should remove the food to be dealt with by a JP and inform the person in charge of the food of his intention.

Any person who might be liable to a prosecution is entitled to be heard and call witnesses. If the JP decides the food does not comply, he will condemn the food and order the food to be destroyed. Any costs incurred will be borne by the owner of the food.

If the notice is withdrawn or the JP refuses to condemn the food, the food authority will pay compensation to the owner of the food. Any dispute to the right or amount of compensation will be determined by arbitration. See Codes of Practice No. 4.

SECTION 10

Improvement Notices: If an officer believes that the proprietor of a food business is failing to comply with any regulations he may be served by an Improvement Notice.

The Improvement Notice must:
State the officer's grounds for believing that the proprietor is failing to comply with the regulations;
Specify the matters which constitute the failure to comply;
Specify the steps the proprietor must take in order to comply;
Require the proprietor to take such measures within a period of time (not less than 14 days).

Any person who fails to comply with an Improvement Notice shall be guilty of an offence. See Codes of Practice No. 5.

SECTION 11

Prohibition Orders: If the proprietor of a food business is convicted of an offence and the court is satisfied that a health risk condition is fulfilled, the court may impose the appropriate prohibition:

A prohibition on the use of the premises or equipment;

A prohibition on the use of a process or treatment.

The prohibition may be imposed on the proprietor to prevent him partaking in the management of any food business.

If the prohibition order is made the authority must serve a copy of the order on the proprietor, and in the case of premises and equipment, affix a copy of the order in a conspicuous position on the premises.

Any person who knowingly contravenes such an order is guilty of an offence.

A prohibition order shall cease to have effect if the authority is satisfied measures have been taken to ensure that there is no health risk. The court issues a certificate within three days of being satisfied after application by the proprietor.

An application cannot be made if it is applied for within six months after the making of the prohibition order, or within three months of a previous application.

SECTION 12

Emergency Prohibition Orders: If an officer is satisfied there is a health risk, he may serve an Emergency Prohibition Notice. If the court decides for the proprietor the authority shall compensate him for any loss suffered by him complying with the notice. Any dispute as to the right or amount of compensation will be determined by arbitration.

See Codes of Practice No. 6.

SECTION 13

Emergency Control Orders, where the minister makes the Order.

If it appears to a minister that a commercial operation

with respect to food, food sources or contact material involves or may involve any risk of injury to health, he may by an Emergency Control Order prohibit the carrying out of that operation.

Any person who knowingly contravenes an Emergency Control Order will be guilty of an offence.

The minister has the power to recover from a person any expenses incurred by him, from the person failing to comply with the Emergency Control Order.

Consumer Protection

SECTION 14

SELLING FOOD NOT OF A NATURE, SUBSTANCE OR QUALITY DEMANDED BY THE CUSTOMER
It will be an offence to sell food with a foreign substance in it, or to sell food under another name not asked for by the customer.

SECTION 15

FALSELY DESCRIBING OR PRESENTING FOOD
There is no defence if the description contained an inaccurate statement on the composition of the food.

SECTION 16

FOOD SAFETY AND CONSUMER PROTECTION
The ministers may make regulations for:
Requiring, prohibiting or regulating the composition of food;
Any food for human consumption meeting bacterial microbiological standards;
Requiring, prohibiting or regulating any process or treatment of food;
Securing the observance of hygiene standards;
Imposing requirements or other regulations for the labelling, marking, presenting or advertising of food;
Any other provisions for securing food complies with the Act and protects the interests of consumers.

In making these regulations the ministers shall have regard to the desirability of restricting the use of substances with no nutritional value.

SECTION 17

ENFORCEMENT OF COMMUNITY PROVISIONS
If the European Community calls for particular provisions with respect to food, ministers may make such provisions as they consider necessary.

SECTION 18

SPECIAL PROVISIONS FOR PARTICULAR FOODS: SPECIAL FOODS
The ministers may make regulations to prohibit:
Carrying out a commercial operation with respect to NOVEL foods or food sources. ('NOVEL foods' are any foods not previously used for human consumption in Great Britain, or used to a very limited extent.)
Carrying out of such operations with respect to GENETICALLY modified food or food source. ('GENETICALLY modified' means genes or other genetic material have been altered by means of an artificial technique, or inherited or derived through any number of replications from genetic material that has been modified.)
The importing of any such food.
The ministers may also make regulations:
In relation to milk of any description the minister may prescribe a designation called SPECIAL DESIGNATION.

SECTION 19

REGISTRATION AND LICENSING OF FOOD PREMISES
See Codes of Practice No. 11.

SECTION 20

OFFENCES DUE TO THE FAULT OF ANOTHER PERSON
Both parties may be proceeded against.

SECTION 21

DEFENCE OF DUE DILIGENCE

In any proceedings it will be a defence for the person charged, that he took all reasonable precautions and exercised all due diligence to avoid committing the offence by himself or persons under his control. If charged with an offence under Section 8, 14, 15, if the person neither: *Prepared the food* or *imported the food*, then he will have satisfied the defence of *Due Diligence*, provided that:
The offence was due to the act or default of another person not under his control;
He carried out all checks of the food that were reasonable;
He did not know or suspect at the time, that his act of omission would be an offence;
The alleged offence was not a sale or intended sale under his name or mark.

DO set up a file and a system for recording. Keep all records for at least six months.

SECTION 22

DEFENCE OF PUBLICATION IN THE COURSE OF BUSINESS

Miscellaneous and Supplemental

SECTION 23

PROVISION OF FOOD HYGIENE TRAINING

A food authority may provide training courses in food hygiene for persons who are or who intend to be involved in a food business, whether as an employee or as a proprietor.

The benefits of having trained staff far outweigh any possible costs of training. When staff have received their training, a training record should be kept for 'due diligence'.

At present there are three professional bodies and these are referred to in the consultative document regarding potential courses for mandatory hygiene training requirements, in respect of the powers contained in the Food Safety Act 1990:

The Royal Institute of Environmental Health Officers;
The Royal Institute of Public Health and Hygiene;
The Royal Society of Health.

All provide a 6–7 hour basic food hygiene course with a certificate for successful candidates.

The courses can only be run and organized by registered training centres, and by using recognized training courses your staff will achieve an acceptable standard of food hygiene.

All staff should have a refresher course at least once a year and should be supported with on the job guidance and assistance from managers.

It is considered that this is only the starting-point. In July 1989 the Government earmarked training as a priority and stated that provision would be made for the compulsory training of 'those people who handle food directly'. Draft regulations are still awaited, but please take note that under the Food Safety Act enforcement officers may at any time issue Improvement Notices requiring training to be carried out within a stated period.

SECTION 24

PROVISION FOR THE FACILITIES FOR CLEANING SHELLFISH

A food authority may make available to the public, tanks or other apparatus for the cleaning of shellfish. The tank should not be on, over or under tidal lands below high water mark of ordinary Spring tides, except by approval of the Secretary of State. (Cleaning in relation to shellfish includes subjecting them to any germicidal treatment.)

SECTION 25

ORDERS FOR FACILITATING THE EXERCISE OF FUNCTIONS

Any person who carries on a relevant business should give to the authorized officer any samples of food and give information to the authorized person.

Any authorized person who discloses any information without the previous consent (in writing) of the person carrying on the business shall be guilty of an offence.

SECTION 26

REGULATIONS AND ORDERS: SUPPLEMENTARY PROVISIONS

Regulates for prohibiting any foods or food source or contact material:

Which fail to comply with the regulations;

Where an offence has been committed or would have been committed if it had taken place in Great Britain.

Regulations under this Section may also:

Require persons to keep records and to produce and provide returns, the particulars to be entered on a register, the register to be kept open to the public;

Prescribe the periods for issuing licences and provide any alteration of conditions, cancellation, suspension or revocation of licences;

Provide for appeal to a magistrate's court or to a tribunal against any decision of an enforcement officer or authority;

Prescribe the procedure for the appeal (including costs) against the tribunal's decision.

Regulations under this section or an order under Section 25 may, provided that the offence is triable, include provisions under which a guilty person will be liable to penalties.

Administration and Enforcement

Administration

SECTION 27

APPOINTING A PUBLIC ANALYST AND A DEPUTY TO ACT IN HIS ABSENCE

SECTION 28

FOR THE FOOD AUTHORITY TO PROVIDE FACILITIES FOR MICROBIOLOGICAL EXAMINATION

Sampling and Analysis, Etc.

SECTION 29

PROCUREMENT OF SAMPLES
See Codes of Practice No. 7.

SECTION 30

ANALYSIS OF SAMPLES
See Codes of Practice No. 7.

SECTION 31

REGULATION OF SAMPLING AND ANALYSIS
See Codes of Practice No. 7.

Powers of Entry and Obstruction

SECTION 32

POWERS OF ENTRY
See Codes of Practice No. 2. Legal Matters.

SECTION 33

OBSTRUCTION OF OFFICERS
See Codes of Practice No. 2.

Offences

SECTION 34

TIME LIMITS FOR PROSECUTION
No prosecution for an offence under this Act, which is punishable, shall be begun after the expiry of three years from the commission of the offence, or one year from its discovery by the prosecutor, whichever is the earlier.

SECTION 35

PUNISHMENT OF OFFENCES
If found guilty of an offence under Section 33 (obstruction):
The fine imposed will not exceed level 5 on the standard scale, or imprisonment for a term of three months or both.
A person found guilty of any other offence under this Act shall be liable:
On conviction, a fine or imprisonment for a term not exceeding two years or both;
On summary conviction, a fine not exceeding the relevant amount or imprisonment for a term not exceeding six months or both.
For Sections 7, 8, or 14 = £20,000; in any other case the statutory maximum.

SECTION 36

OFFENCES BY A CORPORATE BODY
Where the offence has been committed by a corporate organization with the consent or instruction or is in any way attributable to any neglect of any director, manager, secretary or any other similar officer, he, as well as the body corporate, shall be guilty of that offence and is liable to be proceeded against.

Appeals

SECTION 37

APPEALS TO A MAGISTRATE'S COURT
If a person is aggrieved by a decision to serve an enforcement order or the refusal to revoke a prohibition order, they may appeal to a magistrate's court.

The procedure for the appeal is by way of Complaint for an Order and the Magistrates Act shall apply.

The periods for appeal are one month from the date on which the notice of the decision was served on the person wanting to appeal, or the period specified in the improvement order, whichever ends the earlier.

The document should state the right of appeal to a magistrate's court, and the period within such an appeal can be brought.

SECTION 38

APPEALS TO CROWN COURT
If the case is dismissed by magistrates, or the court makes a prohibition order or an emergency prohibition order, a person may appeal to the Crown Court.

SECTION 39

APPEALS AGAINST IMPROVEMENT ORDERS
On appealing against an Improvement Order, a court may cancel or affirm the order, and in doing so may modify the original.

The appeal will be regarded as pending until it is finally disposed of, is withdrawn, or is struck out for want of prosecution.

Prosecution (Sections 34–39)
Authorized officers have a right of entry to premises at 'all reasonable hours' (usually meaning when premises are open for business).

A warrant for forcible entry is available if necessary, and they have the powers to inspect, seize and detain records where appropriate.

It is an offence for anybody to intentionally obstruct Enforcement Officers or to provide false or misleading information.

Time limits for prosecution are three years from the committing of the offence or one year after its discovery, whichever is the earlier. Offences may be tried either at a Magistrate's Court or by a jury at a Crown Court. Penalties are:
On indictment in a Crown Court a maximum of two years prison and/or an unlimited fine;
On summary conviction in a Magistrate's Court, a maximum of six months prison and/or a maximum fine of £2,000.

There are exceptions ... under Sections 7, 8 or 14 (see sections on Legislation) the penalties are the same as above, except that the maximum fine at a Magistrate's Court is increased to £20,000.

Miscellaneous and Supplemental

Powers of Ministers

SECTION 40

POWER TO ISSUE CODES OF PRACTICE
See Codes of Practices Nos 1–11.

SECTION 41

POWER TO REQUIRE RETURNS
Every food authority shall send to the minister such reports or returns and give him the information that he may require.

SECTION 42

Default powers: Where the minister is satisfied that:
A food authority has failed to discharge any duty under the Act;
The authority's failure affects the general interests of consumers of food.
He may empower another authority to discharge that duty in place of the one in default.

The decision will be taken after a local enquiry is held and the Local Government Act shall apply.

Protective Provisions

SECTION 43

CONTINUANCE OF REGISTRATION OR LICENCE ON DEATH
On the death of a person who holds the registration for a food business, the registration shall subsist for the benefit of

the deceased's personal representative, his widow or any other member of his family until the end of:
Three months beginning with his death, or
Such longer periods as the authority may allow.

SECTION 44

PROTECTION OF OFFICERS ACTING IN GOOD FAITH

Financial Provisions

SECTION 45

REGULATIONS AS TO CHARGES
Ministers may make regulations authorizing or requiring charges to be made by authorities in respect of enforcing the Act. The amount shall be at the authority's discretion, subject to a maximum and minimum. It will cover different cases and a sum or method to calculate the amount.

SECTION 46

EXPENSES OF AUTHORIZED OFFICERS AND COUNTY COUNCILS
Expenses incurred in sampling, analysis or examination shall be defrayed by that authority.

SECTION 47

REMUNERATION OF TRIBUNAL CHAIRMAN
Parliament shall provide money to the chairman of any tribunal by way of salary or fees. The minister will act with the approval of the Treasury.

Instruments and Documents

SECTION 48

POWERS OF MINISTERS

Powers to make regulations include power to:

Apply with modifications and adaptations that deal with matters being dealt with;

Make different provisions in relation to different cases;

To provide for such exceptions, limitations and conditions and to make such supplementary, incidental, consequential or transitional provisions as they consider necessary.

Any powers are subject to annulment by either House of Parliament.

Before making any order or regulation the minister shall consult with representative organizations likely to be affected.

SECTION 49

FORM AND AUTHENTICATION OF DOCUMENTS

The following shall be in writing:

All documents authorized or required by the Act, made or issued by the food authority;

All notices and applications given or made to an officer.

SECTION 50

SERVICE OF DOCUMENTS

Concerns ways in which documents may be delivered.

Amendments of Other Acts

SECTION 51

CONTAINMENT OF FOOD: EMERGENCY ORDERS

SECTION 52

MARKETS, SUGAR BEET AND COLD STORAGE

Supplemental

SECTION 53

GENERAL INTERPRETATION

SECTION 54

APPLICATION TO CROWN

SECTION 55

WATER SUPPLY: ENGLAND AND WALES

SECTION 56

WATER SUPPLY: SCOTLAND

SECTION 57

SCILLY ISLES AND CHANNEL ISLANDS

SECTION 58

TERRITORIAL WATERS AND THE CONTINENTAL SHELF

SECTION 59

AMENDMENTS, TRANSITIONAL PROVISIONS, SAVINGS AND REPEALS

SECTION 60

SHORT TITLE: THIS ACT MAY BE CITED AS THE FOOD SAFETY ACT 1990, EXTENT AND COMMENCEMENT

CODES OF PRACTICE

Section 40 Food Safety Act 1990

Ministers may issue Codes of Practice to guide food authorities in the execution and enforcement of the Act and any other legislation made under it. The main aim of a Code of Practice is to develop more consistent standards of enforcement. It does not legally bind the authority, but ministers can issue directions to require the food authority to take specific action in order to comply with a Code of Practice. These directions will be enforceable through the courts.

These Codes of Practice are produced for enforcement officers, but will be of interest to caterers in showing how the Food Safety Act 1990 is likely to be enforced.

CODE OF PRACTICE NO. 1

RESPONSIBILITY FOR ENFORCEMENT OF THE FOOD SAFETY ACT 1990

Sets out the functions to be exercised by district and county councils in the non-metropolitan counties when enforcing the Act. It complements the order made by ministers under Section 5 of the Act. For food authorities to set up co-ordinating groups to liaise between the officers of the county councils and those of other districts in that county. Liaison should involve authorized officers, public analysts, food examiners and any other experts needed to advise the authorities on specific issues.

The group functions should include:

Making arrangements for programmed inspections, especially in food manufacturing premises;

Arranging for co-ordinated advice on specific topics to be provided to businesses in the area;

Arranging for the transfer of any complaint and the sample of food that has been received at the offices of one authority but is in fact the responsibility of another;

Supplying information on the names and telephone numbers of individuals dealing with food law in his authority to any other food authorities in the same area;

Providing a channel for the resolution of any difficulties which may arise;

Co-ordinating sampling programmes;

Recommending priorities for enforcement action;

Co-ordinating on taking legal action;

Appointing a specific liaison officer and a deputy;

Dealing with enquiries and complaints by the public.
Enforcement of the Act:
Section 12 enforced by district councils
Section 15 enforced by county councils

All food authorities have a duty to enforce Sections 7, 8 and 14 and take legal proceedings. Responsibilities should be divided thus:

With contamination by micro-organisms or their toxins, e.g. salmonella, listeria or botulism, district councils should investigate and take legal proceedings. County councils should pass any such case to the district council.

In cases of chemical contamination and improper use of additives, the County Council should undertake the routine checks and analysis of food and take legal proceedings. County councils should take account of the possible hygiene or public health implications and draw the attention of the district council for the need of a hygiene inspection.

For contamination by mould or foreign matter, district councils should investigate and take legal proceedings. They should liaise with other authorities, and if malicious tampering is suspected they should also contact the police.

CODE OF PRACTICE No. 2

LEGAL MATTERS

The handling of consumer complaints:
If preliminary enquiries suggest that the complaint may well be founded, the food authority should inform the supplier, manufacturer or importer. Initial notification may be oral but should be followed by written notification containing the date and nature of the complaint. If malicious contamination is suspected the food authority should liaise with the police.
Investigation of complaint samples: If the food authority declares the complaint sample should be analysed he has certain steps to take:
That the sample should be analysed by a person suitably qualified;
That the sample is properly stored and handled;
Powers of entry;
All covered by Sections 32–3 Food Safety Act.
Prosecutions should be brought without delay. In England

and Wales all legal proceedings are subject to the requirements of the Police and Criminal Evidence Act 1984 and Codes of Practice under Section 66 of that Act. Reference should be made to those especially in relation to the procedures for gathering evidence.

CODE OF PRACTICE NO. 3

INSPECTION PROCEDURES

Inspection means a visit to any food premises for the purpose of one of the following:
Inspection of premises;
Inspection of equipment (including cleaning and maintenance);
Inspection of a process;
Inspection of the hygiene practices of the staff;
Inspection of the food;
Inspection of labels and advertising material;
and/or
Inspection of records.

It does not mean a visit solely to deal with complaints, or visits to advise traders who have requested information, or a visit solely to obtain samples, or a visit to ensure compliance with an improvement order, or to check before prosecution, or conducting a survey.

As a general rule, inspections will be made without prior warning. After inspection an officer should report in writing to the owner of the business. The report should state:
The date, time and place of the inspection;
What was examined;
Whether any samples were taken;
The officer's conclusions.

In some circumstances the report will take a specified form, e.g. an Improvement Order.

CODE OF PRACTICE NO. 4

INSPECTION, DETENTION AND SEIZURE OF SUSPECT FOOD

Section 9 of the Act.

Powers of Entry, Sections 32–3 and the Code of Practice No. 2 cover this Code.

When to use detention and seizure powers:
If food fails to comply with Food Safety requirements, as in Section 8 the officer may detain and seize the food. Section 9; If possible the food should be brought before a JP to be dealt with within eight days. In the case of highly perishable foods, the case should be dealt with within two days.

Detention of food:
In the event of a food poisoning outbreak, the officer should seek expert advice from the consultant in Communicable Disease Control and may need to contact the local Public Health Laboratory Service. Wherever possible and appropriate there should be full and open discussions with the owner or the person in charge of the food and with the manufacturer.

Giving notice of seizure or detention:
The decision to detain or seize food should only be taken by appropriately qualified officers. When food is seized, written confirmation of the seizure must be given immediately.

The detention of food notice should only be signed by the officer detaining the food. Officers who deliver the notice need not hold the same qualifications as the detaining officer but should be able to explain the purpose of the notice and deal with any difficulties, e.g. obstruction.

Seizure of food:
The officer should have regard to the chain of evidence, where this might be crucial in any subsequent prosecution and should not leave the food unattended. If he is confident the food will not be removed, or used for human consumption, or the evidence destroyed, he may leave it, but the officers will be required to prove that the food produced before the JP is the food that was seized.

Methods of service of notice:
The notice used in the enforcement of Section 9 should be served by hand on the person in charge of the food, and by courtesy also notify the owner of the food. Up to two days can be allowed for having this dealt with by a JP and to allow witnesses to be contacted.

Withdrawal of notice of detention:
The decision to issue a withdrawal of detention of food notice should be taken by the officer who originally issued the notice. This should be served as soon as possible.

Taking action without inspecting:
The provisions of Section 9 apply equally to food which has not been inspected. This would occur when it appears to the officer the food is so contaminated or that it is likely to cause food poisoning or any disease communicable to human beings.

Dealing with batches, lots of consignments of food:
All covered by Sections 8–9.

Unco-operative proprietors:
All covered by Sections 32–3.

Compensation: Section 9
Voluntary procedures:
Where food is voluntarily surrendered for destruction a receipt should be issued and the description of the food should include 'voluntarily surrendered for destruction'. The receipt should be signed by the person surrendering the food.

Appearance before a justice of the peace:
See methods of serving a notice.

Destruction or Disposal of food:
The food authority will be responsible for oganizing the destruction or disposal of food, and arrangements should be made for the food to be fully supervised until it can be dealt with. It should be destroyed by total destruction, e.g. incineration. If that is not possible by e.g. flattening tin cans for disposal, then by any method to ensure there is no possibility of the food returning to the food chain.

CODE OF PRACTICE NO. 5

THE USE OF IMPROVEMENT ORDERS
When to use an improvement order. Section 10.

An Improvement Notice should only be served when the officer is confident there is no imminent risk to health. See Code of Practice No. 6 Prohibition procedures. The use of an Improvement Order should be used as the first option where defects are found on inspection.

Who should issue an Improvement Notice:
Only a fully qualified officer with experience in food law enforcement.

Service of the Notice:
The Act requires the notice to be served on the proprietor.

Drafting the Notice:
It is important that the receipient of the notice knows what is wrong and why it is wrong. Therefore the wording of the notice should be clear and easily understood. It is not sufficient to simply quote the Act.

Time to be specified on the Notice:
The Improvement Notice should clearly specify the measures to be taken, and the period of time within which the proprietor must complete the measures. The minimum period which may be specified is fourteen days and the period for completing the work should be a realistic one.

Requests for extensions of time:
There is no specific provision in the Food Safety Act to extend the time limit on a notice, but if an officer considers a request for an extension of a time limit is reasonable, he may decide not to enforce the notice straightaway.

Appeals
See Section 39.

Compliance:
To maintain good working relationships the officer should, if possible, liaise with the proprietor while the work is being done and encourage the proprietor to notify the authority when the work is done. When the work is completed, the work should be checked.

CODE OF PRACTICE NO. 6

PROHIBITION PROCEDURES (SECTION 11, 12 FOOD SAFETY ACT)

This covers the consideration of prohibition, whereby the authorized officer should use professional judgement to decide whether a premises, a process, a treatment or a piece of equipment, or its use involves an imminent risk to health.

Conditions where prohibition of premises may be appropriate:

Serious infestation by rats, mice, cockroaches or other vermin, including birds, or a combination of these infestations, resulting in actual food contamination or a real risk of food contamination.

Very poor structural condition and poor equipment and/or poor maintenance of routine cleaning, and/or serious accumulations of refuse, filth or other extraneous matter resulting in a real risk of food contamination.

Serious drainage defects or flooding of premises.

Premises or practices which seriously contravene the Food Hygiene (General) Regulations 1970 and have been, or are, involved with an outbreak of food poisoning.

Any combination of the above which together represent an imminent risk of injury to health.

Conditions where prohibition of equipment may be appropriate:

In addition to the above:

Use of defective equipment e.g. a pasteurizer incapable of achieving the required pasteurizing temperature.

The use of equipment involving high-risk foods which has been inadequately cleaned or disinfected or is obviously grossly contaminated and can no longer be properly cleaned.

Conditions where prohibition of a process may be appropriate:

Serious risk of cross contamination.

Inadequate temperature control, e.g. failure to achieve a high enough cooking temperature.

Operation outside critical control criteria, e.g. incorrect pH

of a product that might allow clostridium botulinum to multiply.
The use of a process for a product to which it is inappropriate.

CODE OF PRACTICE NO. 7

SAMPLING FOR ANALYSIS OR EXAMINATION

This relates to the procedure which authorized officers should follow when procuring and handling food samples.

Analysis is defined as including microbiological assay and any technique to determine the composition of food.

Examination is defined as solely relating to microbiological examination.

Samples for analysis should only be taken by authorized officers who are properly trained in the appropriate techniques. All such officers should be suitably qualified or experienced in food law enforcement.

The formal sample should be divided into three. Where practicable the division should be carried out on the premises of the seller/owner of the food. They should be placed in clean, dry, leakproof containers secured with a tamper-evident seal and labelled with the name of the food; the name of the officer; the name of the authority; the place, date, and time of sampling, and an identification number.

Samples for examination need not be divided into three, since the distribution of bacterial contaminants means no two samples will be the same.

If it is decided an alleged offence has taken place, the manufacturer and the owner of the food should be informed immediately by the fastest, possible means, e.g. fax or telephone, then confirmed in writing. Any person so notified is entitled, on request, to a copy of the certificate of examination.

CODE OF PRACTICE NO. 8

FOOD STANDARDS INSPECTION

The purpose of a food standards inspection is to ensure food standards are being met.

Food standards means legal requirements covering the

quality, composition, labelling, presentation and advertising of food.

Premises assessed to present a high risk to food standards should be inspected at least once a year, medium risk every two years and low risk every five years.

CODE OF PRACTICE NO. 9

FOOD HYGIENE INSPECTION

A food hygiene inspection has two main purposes:
Authorized officers should identify contraventions of the Food Safety Act 1990 and food hygiene and food processing regulations and seek to have them corrected.
Authorized officers should seek to identify potential risks arising from the activities carried on, such as processing, cooking, handling and storage of food.
Wherever it is practicable and appropriate to do so a food hygiene inspection should be combined with:
A food standards inspection;
An inspection carried out under other legislation and/or
Another visit for food hygiene purposes.
A letter should be sent after the visit stating:
A report of a food hygiene inspection carried out under the Food Safety Act 1990.

CODE OF PRACTICE NO. 10

ENFORCEMENT OF THE TEMPERATURE CONTROL REQUIREMENTS OF THE FOOD HYGIENE REGULATIONS

CODE OF PRACTICE NO. 11

ENFORCEMENT OF THE FOOD PREMISES REGISTRATION REGULATIONS

CODE OF PRACTICE NO. 12

DIVISION OF ENFORCEMENT RESPONSIBILITIES FOR THE QUICK FROZEN FOODSTUFF REGULATIONS 1990

This regulation came into force on 10 January 1991. 'Quick frozen' foodstuff does not include ice-cream or any other edible ice.

These regulations do not apply to any food:
That is intended for sale for human consumption;
Which is supplied under Government contracts for consumption by HM Forces or supplied for consumption by a visiting Force.
The food should be labelled 'quick frozen'.

CODE OF PRACTICE NO. 13

ENFORCEMENT OF THE FOOD SAFETY ACT 1990 IN RELATION TO CROWN PREMISES

Crown premises fall into 2 groups:
Category 1: Includes premises situated on Crown Land, but where there are no problems of security, e.g. restaurants in museums or Royal Parks. These premises can be treated like any other food business.
Category 2: Those premises with entry requirements, but only a slight security risk. Most Government buildings fall into this category. They are similar to many private businesses with security systems.
Category 3: Those where unannounced entry is not possible because of serious security implications and/or for the personal safety of the authorized officer, e.g. official residences of the Royal Family and senior members of the Government, all MOD establishments, prisons and remand centres, and those parts of police premises where prisoners are or may be detained.
The provisions of the Act apply to people in the public service of the Crown as they apply to other people, but they do not apply to:
Her Majesty the Queen or His Royal Highness the Prince of Wales as private individuals;
Premises occupied by them in their private capacities, e.g. Balmoral, Sandringham or Highgrove.
The Act does not allow the Crown to be prosecuted.

The Secretary of State will issue certificates that state that, in the interest of national security, the powers of entry under the Act cannot be exercised.

FOOD HYGIENE (GENERAL) REGULATIONS 1970

REGULATION 1: DEFINITION OF FOOD

REGULATION 2: SALE OF FOOD

REGULATION 3: FOOD FOR HUMAN CONSUMPTION

REGULATION 4: DEFINES MINISTERS' POWERS

REGULATION 5: ENFORCEMENT

REGULATION 6: INSANITARY PREMISES

A food business must not be carried on in any premises where the situation, condition or construction is such that food is exposed to the risk of contamination. Insanitary premises will include those infested with pests, with defective or leaking drains, or where there is such a lack of cleaning that the premises are filthy. Also includes premises which are not easy to keep clean and hygienic because of their poor structural condition.

A breach of this regulation is likely to result in the issue of an Emergency Prohibition Notice (Section 12 Food Safety Act).

REGULATION 7: ARTICLES AND EQUIPMENT

Equipment must not be made of absorbent material, such as wood, and must be kept clean and in good condition.

REGULATION 8: DOMESTIC PREMISES

Caterers are restricted by law on the use of domestic premises for catering purposes. They cannot allow any food to be prepared or packed by any person in domestic premises where the food will subsequently be sold from the caterer's premises.

This regulation allows an exemption (subject to certain conditions) where the food given out is shrimps or prawns for peeling on domestic premises. But, as other regulations apply, if you intend to use domestic premises for catering purposes of any kind, you will be well advised to contact your local EHO for his advice and guidance, and to check your premises for suitability for use.

REGULATION 9: PROTECTION FROM RISK OF CONTAMINATION

A food handler must take all reasonable precautions to protect food from the risk of contamination.

Ensure food unfit for human consumption be kept away from clean food and labelled as unfit.

In an outside yard or forecourt, food must be placed no lower than 48 cm from the ground (unless adequately protected).

Open food must (where reasonably necessary) be kept covered or screened from possible contamination when exposed for sale (during sale or delivery). Closed display cabinets and sneeze guards meet this requirement.

'Where reasonably necessary' means in some cases no screening is required.

Consideration needs to be given to:

The type of food to be displayed. Is it high risk? Will it support the growth of bacteria?

The length of time the food is on display;

The temperature control of the food on display;

Likely sources and types of contamination.

Animal foods must not be kept in any food room unless in a closed container so that it cannot contaminate any food in that room.

REGULATION 10: PERSONAL CLEANLINESS

Food handlers must:

Keep all parts of the body likely to come into contact with food as clean as possible;

Wear clean protective clothing;

Cover cuts and sores with a waterproof dressing;

Not spit;

Not smoke in any food room;

Report any illness to their employers.

REGULATION 11: PROTECTIVE CLOTHING

Food handlers must at all times wear clean protective clothing to protect the food from the bacteria present on the person.
This applies to all food handlers with a few exceptions:
Those who only handle raw vegetables and intoxicating liquor and soft drinks. (Thus bar staff are exempt as long as they *only* serve drinks and packaged goods, e.g. crisps, nuts. If they also serve meals and snacks they must comply.)
Waiters in a catering business;
Persons only engaged in carrying unskinned rabbits, hares or unplucked game and poultry;
In transporting food by rail or by any other carrier where the vehicle used does not normally carry food.
The exceptions apply provided the person carrying the food takes all precautions to prevent the food coming into contact with any exposed part of the body, or their clothing. Any food handler carrying meat (which is open food) that is liable to come into contact with their head or neck, must wear clean and washable head and neck coverings. Hair must be covered with a suitable covering which prevents hair falling into food.

REGULATION 12: CARRIAGE AND WRAPPING OF FOOD

Food handlers must not carry any food in a container together with any article that may contaminate the food, or with any live animal or poultry. Materials used for wrapping the food must be clean and not contaminate the food. The only printed material that is allowed to come into contact with open food is material specifically designed for food wrapping.
Exemptions: raw vegetables, unskinned rabbits, hares or unplucked game and poultry.

REGULATION 13: PERSONS SUFFERING FROM CERTAIN INFECTIONS

If the food handlers become aware they are suffering from (or a carrier of) any of the infections listed below, they should inform their employer:

Typhoid fever
Paratyphoid fever
Salmonella infections
Amoebic dysentery
Bacilliary dysentery
Any staphylococcus infection (septic cuts, boils, throat or nose infections).

REGULATION 14: SOIL DRAINAGE SYSTEM

REGULATION 15: CISTERNS FOR SUPPLYING WATER TO A FOOD ROOM

REGULATION 16: SANITARY CONVENIENCES

Sanitary conveniences situated in, or regularly used by any food handler, must be kept clean and well maintained. They should be positioned so that no offensive odour can penetrate into any food room. The room containing the toilet must be kept clean and properly lighted and ventilated. No food, articles or equipment, likely to come into contact with food, may be kept in any room containing a sanitary convenience.

No food room which connects directly with a room containing a sanitary convenience can be used for the handling of open food.

Under the Health and Safety at Work Act 1974, there must be an intervening, ventilated space between any room containing a sanitary convenience and a food room.

A clearly legible notice requesting food handlers to 'wash your hands' must be fixed in a prominent position near every toilet used by them.

REGULATION 17: WATER SUPPLY

A water supply, sufficient in quantity to enable these regulations to be complied with, must be provided at all food premises. The supply must be clean and wholesome and must normally be constant.

REGULATION 18: WASHHAND BASINS

All food premises must have suitable and sufficient washhand basins for the use of food handlers, placed in the premises and in conveniently accessible positions.
There should be an adequate supply of hot and cold water, or hot water at a suitably controlled temperature.
There must be soap or a suitable detergent available in dispensers and the type of soap chosen should be suitable for the water in the district.
Nail-brushes should be provided and suitable drying facilities at each washhand basin.
Communal roller towels should not be used as they present a serious danger in transferring bacteria.
Every washhand basin must be kept clean and in good working condition.
Washhand basins must only be used for food handlers to wash their hands.

REGULATION 19: FIRST-AID BOX

Businesses must supply first-aid materials, to comply with the Food Safety Act. There must be a sufficient supply of waterproof dressings of a distinctive colour for first-aid treatment, they must be provided at the food premises and must be readily available to the food handler. To comply with the Health and Safety at Work Act 1979 you will need:
3 packs of 14 sterile dressings (of a distinctive colour)
8 sterile medium dressings (No. 8)
4 sterile large dressings (No. 9)
4 sterile extra large dressings (No. 3)
4 sterile large pads (No. 16)
4 sterile triangular bandages
2 bunches of 6 safety pins
100 g pack of cotton wool
2 or 3 melolin dressings
1 micropore surgical tape
3 pairs disposable gloves
3 disposable bags
1 plastic apron
1 leaflet on advice for first-aid treatment

REGULATION 20: STORAGE OF OUTDOOR CLOTHING

No personal effects are permitted in the food area.

REGULATION 21: FACILITIES FOR WASHING FOOD AND EQUIPMENT

There shall be provided in all food premises, where open food is handled, sinks or other washing facilities suitable and sufficient for any necessary washing of food and equipment used in the food business.
Reference to a sink includes any other suitable washing facility.
Every sink shall have an adequate supply of hot and cold water, or hot water at a suitably controlled temperature, or cold water where the sink is used:
Only for washing fish, fruit or vegetables; or for washing with a suitable bactricidal agent only, drinking vessels, or only, ice-cream formers or servers.
Every sink shall be kept clean and in good working condition.

REGULATION 22: LIGHTING OF FOOD ROOMS

Suitable and sufficient means of lighting shall be provided in every food room and every such room shall be suitably and sufficiently lighted.

REGULATION 23: VENTILATION OF FOOD ROOMS

Except in the case of a room in which the humidity or temperature is controlled, suitable and sufficient means of ventilation shall be provided in every food room and suitable and sufficient ventilation shall be maintained there.

REGULATION 24: FOOD ROOM NOT TO BE USED AS A SLEEPING PLACE

REGULATION 25: CLEANLINESS AND REPAIR OF FOOD ROOMS

The walls, floors, door, windows, ceiling, woodwork and all other parts of the structure of any food room shall be kept clean and be kept in such good order, repair and conditions as to enable them to be effectively cleaned; and prevent, so far as is reasonably practicable, the entry of birds, and any risk of infestation by rats, mice, insects or other pests.

REGULATION 26: ACCUMULATION OF REFUSE

The layout of premises must provide adequate space suitably sited for the removal of waste from food, for the separation of unfit food and the storage of waste or unfit food prior to disposal.

Refuse or filth, whether solid or liquid, must not be deposited or allowed to accumulate in a food room except (so far as may be unavoidable) for the proper carrying on of the business.

Refuse awaiting disposal should not be stored for too long. Short term storage in a properly constructed, lidded container may be allowed in a kitchen, provided that at the end of the preparation or service period the contents are removed to the designated storage area.

REGULATION 27: TEMPERATURE CONTROL

See Food Hygiene (Amendment) Regulations 1990.

REGULATION 28: EXEMPTION OF PERSONS FROM CERTAIN REQUIREMENTS

REGULATION 29: OFFENCES

See Food Safety Act 1990.

REGULATION 30: PENALTIES

See Food Safety Act 1990.

FOOD HYGIENE (AMENDMENT) REGULATIONS 1990

SECTION 1

Relevant foods, temperature, exemptions and exceptions. See following temperature controls.

SECTION 2

Temperatures and start dates.

See following temperature controls. Three temperatures are specified: two for chill foods (8°C and 5°C) and one for hot food (63°C).

Three dates are also specified:

From 1 April 1991 all relevant foods kept below 5°C or above 63°C (includes delivery vehicles over 7.5 tonnes, excludes small vehicles making local deliveries);

From 1 April 1992 includes small vehicles;

From 1 May 1993 subset of foods maintained below 5°C.

Exemptions:

Small delivery vehicles for no longer than twelve hours;

Maximum allowable chill temperature 8°C;

Hot allowable temperature above 63°C.

SECTION 3

Exclusions and exemptions.

SECTION 4

Compliance implications.

Temperature controls and recording

Chill foods

Monitoring and measuring temperatures

Using non-destructive measurement

Food probing

See temperature controls.

SECTION 5

Other minor provisions.

Maximum Temperatures at which Different Foods must be Stored

FOOD	DATE AND TEMP. From 1 April 1991	From 1 April 1993
CHEESE		
Uncut or whole mould ripened soft cheese. e.g. Brie, Danish Blue, Stilton, Roquefort, Camembert, Dolcelatte. (These temperatures apply only when the cheese is ripened.)	8°C	8°C
The cut segment of above.	8°C	5°C
The remaining portion of above included in a cooked product, intended for further heating before consumption.	8°C	8°C
Hard and soft cheese included in a cooked product intended to be eaten without further reheating.	8°C	5°C
Hard cheeses not contained in a cooked product; cream or curd cheese, cottage cheese.	Not covered in these regs.	
Unripened soft cheese.	Not covered in these regs.	
COOKED PRODUCTS		
Containing meat, fish, eggs (or their substitutes) hard and soft cheese, cereals, pulses, vegetables.	8°C	5°C
Cooked products intended to be eaten without further reheating:		
Cooked poultry and cold cooked meats – ham, tongue, corned beef, luncheon meat (once removed from the can).	8°C	5°C
Cooked vegetable or cereal salads, e.g. potato, rice, cooked bean salads.	8°C	5°C

FOOD	DATE AND TEMP. From 1 April 1991	From 1 April 1993
Meat and fish pate, e.g. Brussels, Ardennes, smoked mackerel pâté.	8°C	5°C
Scotch eggs, pork pies with gelatine added after cooking.	8°C	5°C
Quiches, open- or lattice-topped savoury pies. Sandwich fillings (see exemption on made up sandwiches), e.g. chicken, cold cooked sausages, egg mayonnaise, tuna, made-up mixtures of relevant foods.	8°C	5°C
Where manufacturer's instructions need reheating, e.g. certain meat, fish or chicken pies, pizza, many ready-made meals.	8°C	5°C
Cooked sausage rolls to be sold on the day of their production or the next day.	Not covered	
Cooked pies and pasties containing meat, fish or substitutes, or vegetables in pastry, with nothing added to them, e.g. gelatine, to be sold on the day of their production or the next day.	Not covered	
SMOKED OR CURED FISH		
Whether whole or cut/sliced after smoking or curing, e.g. smoked salmon, smoked mackeral, smoked trout, smoked haddock, kippers.	8°C	5°C

FOOD	DATE AND TEMP. From 1 April 1991	From 1 April 1993
SMOKED OR CURED MEAT		
When cut/sliced after smoking or curing, e.g. cured cooked ham, salamis, other fermented (continental style) sausages.	8°C	5°C
DAIRY-BASED DESSERTS (INCLUDING MILK SUBSTITUTES)		
With a pH value of 4.5 or more, e.g. fromage frais, mousses, creme caramels, whipped cream desserts.	8°C	8°C
With a pH value under 4.5 e.g. most yoghurts	Not covered	
PREPARED VEGETABLE SALADS		
Including those containing fruit, e.g. coleslaws and prepared fresh vegetable salads.	8°C	8°C
Prepared salads which contain foods subject to 5°C such as rice salad.	8°C	5°C
UNCOOKED OR PARTLY COOKED PASTRY AND DOUGH PRODUCTS		
Containing meat, fish or substitutes, e.g. uncooked or partly cooked pizzas, sausage rolls, fresh pasta with meat or fish filling, e.g. ravioli.	8°C	8°C
SANDWICHES, FILLED ROLLS AND BREAD PRODUCTS		
Containing ripened soft cheese, smoked or cured fish or cut or sliced smoked or cured meat, other cooked products not intended to be sold within twenty-four hours of preparation.	8°C	5°C
As above but intended to be sold within twenty-four hours of preparation.	8°C	8°C

Containing hard cheese not mixed with any other relevant foods, e.g. lettuce, tomato.	Not covered	
Cold sandwiches to be sold within four hours of completion of preparation.	Not covered	
DAIRY CREAM CAKES Excludes non-dairy cream cakes	8°C	8°C

ALL THE FOLLOWING ARE NOT COVERED:

Fruit pies

Bread, biscuits, cakes or pastry (which would be covered by the regulations only because they contain egg or milk before baking)

Uncooked bacon and uncooked ham, including Parma ham, Bayonne ham or uncooked smoked bacon

Dry pasta, dry pudding mixes or dry mixes for the preparation of beverages

Chocolate or sugar confectionary

Milk, including separated or skimmed milk, dried milk, condensed milk and cream (when not combined with other ingredients)

Preserved foods, e.g. dried vegetables, packet soups, pickled foods, preserves and jams

Foods preserved by a process of heating and packed in hermetically sealed containers whilst still in the container, e.g. canned foods, long life soup.

RETAIL AND CATERING EXEMPTIONS

These regulations do not apply to relevant foods in the following circumstances:

If they are in a food room and are intended to be sold within two hours of the conclusion of preparation and are kept at 63°C or above.

If they are in a food room and are intended to be sold within four hours of the conclusion of preparation and are kept at a temperature below 63°C.

Relevant food displayed for up to four hours to allow for self-service displays, buffets, sweet trolley and cheese boards, but no more food than is reasonably necessary for display or service at any one time.

Specified temperatures (63°C and 5°C–8°C) may be exceeded by 2°C for not more than two hours under the following circumstances:

During preparation of food;

While defrosting food;

During temporary breakdown of equipment;

During movement of food from one part of the premises to another.

These regulations do seem complicated but the overall aim is simple – to prevent the multiplication of spoilage and food poisoning bacteria in vulnerable foods.

7 Record Keeping

The owner of the business is the person ultimately responsible for the proper standards of hygiene, safety and food composition. He can delegate that responsibility to another person, e.g. a manager or supervisor who should carry on the business to the instructions of the owner. In the case of a prosecution it may well be the owner of the business who is taken to court. But if he can prove the offence was due to fault of another, he can prove the defence of 'due diligence'.

The following forms are intended as an example of records to be kept in order to help a defendant and food traders who may be taken to court by the local Food Authority. They can also be shown to an EHO on a routine visit to show that the owner of the business is taking care and will help to prove to a court that he has taken all reasonable precautions and exercised 'due diligence'.

A court will scrutinize the methods used to record and secure proper standards whenever 'due diligence' is claimed.

Use a temperature control sheet daily to record temperatures of food being stored prior to service.

Use a cleaning schedule to show that there is attention to detail and that cleaning is being carried out on a regular basis.

Use a hygiene inspection sheet to carry out your own inspection.

Record Keeping

The forms included cover:
Temperature Monitoring
Pre-employment Questionnaire

Review Health Screening
Hygiene and Health and Safety Training
Customer Complaint Record
Food Hazard Warning
Delivery Monitoring
Pest Control Record
Cleaning Schedule
Health and Safety Data for Chemicals Used
Hygiene Inspection For Retail Premises
Accident Book

Temperature Monitoring

Week ending______________ Signed________________

	Sun.	Mon.	Tues.	Wed.	Thurs.	Fri.	Sat.
Unit No.							
Chilled							
Chilled							
Chilled							
Freezer							
Freezer							
Freezer							
Hot Display							
Hot Display							

Action taken if temperature exceeds tolerances __________

____

Signed ________________

Pre-Employment Questionnaire

For all catering staff and food handlers:

Name ____________________ Date of birth ____________

Address __________________ Telephone ______________

Name and address of doctor ___________________________

____

Have you ever had any of the following?	If Yes HOW LONG OFF WORK	DOCTOR HOSPITAL
Typhoid, paratyphoid or eneteric fevers?		Y/N
Food poisoning?		Y/N
Dysentery?		Y/N
Persistent diarrhoea or bowel infection?		Y/N
Tuberculosis?		Y/N
Any tropical disease?		Y/N

Have you had any of the following over the last two years?

Chronic Bronchitis?	Y/N
Diarrhoea and/or vomiting for more than two days?	Y/N
Skin rash/skin disease?	Y/N
Recurrent boils/septic cuts?	Y/N
Discharge from ear, eye, nose?	Y/N
Have you lived abroad in the last ten years?	Y/N
Have you been abroad in the last two years?	Y/N

If yes where and when?

I declare that all of the above statements are true to the best of my knowledge and belief.

Signed ____________________ Date ____________________

Review Health Screening

To be completed by all catering staff on return to work after absence due to illness, injury or holidays abroad.

Name of employee ______________________________

Address ______________________________

____

Telephone ______________________________

Holiday abroad, countries visited ______________________________

Have you suffered from sickness, diarrhoea or any stomach disorder? Y/N

Have you had any 'flu-like' symptoms in the last forty-eight hours? Y/N

Have you had any contact with anyone with typhoid, paratyphoid, cholera, dysentery, salmonellae infections, gastro-enteritis, sickness or diarrhoea? Y/N

Are you suffering from any infections of the skin, nose, throat, eyes or ears? Y/N

Have you suffered any of these conditions since you have been away from work? Y/N

Signature of employee ______________________________

Signature of supervisor/manager ______________________________

Date ______________________________

Hygiene and Health and Safety Training Record

Name	Induction	Job	Tasks	Basic food hygiene	Cleaning techniques	Intermediate hygiene	Advanced hygiene	Health & Safety training

Customer Complaint Record

Date ____________ Time __________ Unit __________

Received by: ____

Customer's Name ____________________________________

Address ____

____

Telephone ____

Food subject to complaint ____________________________

Nature of complaint _________________________________

Money refunded? (Attach till refund slip) _____________

Product bought in? *Y/N* *Our own product?* *Y/N*

Supplier _________________ Ingredients ______________

Manufacturer _____________ Chef ___________________

Attach copies of delivery note, temperature records, coding checks etc.

Any deficiences noted in records? Y/N.
If Yes give details ___________________________________

Action taken ____

Signed ___________________ Date __________________

Food Hazard Warning

Date ____________________ Time ____________________

Information received from ____________________

The following food has been notified as:

Trade withdrawal
Food Hazard Warning
Emergency control order

Type of food ____________________

Brand name ____________________

Manufacturer ____________________

Country of origin ____________________

Importer/distributer ____________________

Code/other mark ____________________

Pack weight/size ____________________

Reason for action ____________________

No further deliveries of this product are to be accepted until this notice is withdrawn.

Action taken if stock already
on the premises ____________________

Signed ____________________ Date ____________________

Delivery Monitoring

Delivery date ____________ Delivery time __________

Received by ____________________________________

Product ________________ Supplier ____________

Vehicle Reg. No. _______

Despatch temperature ___________________________

Delivery temperature ____________________________

Use by date ______________________________________

Any visible damage? _____________________________

Accept or reject? Reasons _________________________

Signed _________________ Date _________________

Pest Control Record

Report

Date ____________ Time ____________ Unit ____________

Problem ____

Pests seen/identified? ________________________________

Location ____

Reported by ______________ Department ______________

Action ____

Date investigated ____________ Time investigated ________

Pests identified ____________________________________

Action taken ______________________________________

Signature of pest control operator ______________________

Date ____

Comments ______________________________________

Cleaning Schedule

Week ending ______________________________

Completed by	Task	Mon.	Tues.	Wed.	Thurs.	Fri.	Sat.	Sun.	Checked by
	Work surfaces								
	Chopping-boards								
	Equipment								
	Utensils								
	Fridges								
	Freezers								
	Chillers								
	Prep. sinks								
	Grills, ovens								
	Cooking range								
	Microwaves								
	Deep fat fryers								
	Extractors								
	Washing-up sink								
	Crockery								
	Waste bins and stands								
	Shelving, doors, walls								
	Dispense equipment								
	Handwash area								
	Floors								

Health and Safety Data for Chemicals Used

PRODUCT

Description ______________________________

PHYSICAL PROPERTIES

Boiling point ______________________________

Specific gravity ______________________________

COMPOSITION

SUPPLY LABEL

Classification ______________________________

Hazard symbol ______________________________

Risk phases ______________________________

Safety phases ______________________________

STORAGE AND HANDLING

Personal ______________________________

Storage conditions ______________________________

Fire hazard ______________________________

Disposal ______________________________

EMERGENCY MEASURES

Spillage ______________________________

First aid: skin, eyes, ingestion, inhalation ______________

Additional information ______________________________

Hygiene Inspection for Retail Premises

These are guidelines for carrying out a hygiene inspection for premises where food is sold.

1 GENERAL ASSESSMENT OF PROCEDURES
Are there any documentation or records that will assist in the inspection?
Are there any high-risk areas in the premises that require particular attention?

2 MANAGEMENT PROCEDURES
Does the manager know about high risk foods and quality assurance?
Are any particular food hazards identified and evaluated?
Is this appropriate?
What hazards exist?
Are the critical control points (CCPs) identified?
Is there an effective product recall procedure?

3 PREMISES
Are the floors of suitable construction?
Are the walls of appropriate construction?
Are the doors of appropriate construction and close-fitting?
Is adequate lighting provided in the food handling area?
Are the standards of cleanliness of the structure acceptable?

FACILITIES

4 PREPARATION OF SURFACES
Are the preparation areas adequate to prevent cross contamination?
Are the surfaces impervious, in good order and condition to enable them to be readily cleaned?

5 PREPARATION SINKS

Are there hot and cold water supplies to the sink?
Are the supplies adequate for the business?
Are there sufficient sinks for the size of the business?
Is there a separate sink for washing equipment?
Are the sinks in good order?

6 HANDWASHING FACILITIES

Are they accessible in suitable locations and adequate for the purpose?
Are they provided with hot and cold water?

7 SANITATION

Are the toilets adequate for the number of staff?
Are the toilets clean?
Does the location pose any risk of contamination to the food?

8 FIRST AID

Is a first-aid kit readily available?
Are the contents adequate?
Does the kit contain waterproof dressings of a distinctive colour?

9 CLOTHING AND STORAGE

Is outdoor clothing stored away from open food?
If lockers are provided are they:
- durable?
- easily cleaned?
- adequately ventilated?

10 WATER SUPPLY

Is the water used direct from the mains or from a storage tank?
Is the tank adequately protected at all times from any form of contamination?
Is the microbiological quality of the water supply suitable?

11 TEMPERATURE

Are relevant cooked or ready-to-eat foods displayed or stored under refrigeration temperatures?

Are the chilled and frozen food refrigeration units maintaining the required temperatures?
Are the chilled and frozen food units regularly maintained and serviced?
Are temperature indicating thermometers provided and are they operating?
Is there a system of temperature monitoring in operation?
Are records of operating temperatures retained?

12 FOOD HANDLING TECHNIQUES AND PRACTICES

Are separate areas of the premises used for raw and cooked foods?
Are raw and cooked foods stored properly when in refrigerators, freezers or in display cabinets?
Are separate refrigerators provided?
Is open cooked food protected from contamination?
Are separate slicers provided and used? Is the cleaning adequate and at appropriate intervals?
Are different members of staff handling raw and cooked foods?
Are the chopping-boards in good condition? Is there evidence of old stock?
Are foods being stored under suitable conditions and in accordance with instructions?
Is there evidence of excessive damage to food cartons or containers?

13 FOOD HANDLERS

Is there any evidence of poor food hygiene practices?
Do staff wash their hands before handling food, after visiting the toilets and after handling raw foods?
Are cuts, sores and abrasions left uncovered?
Are staff smoking or using tobacco, or eating in the food room?
Are the staff handling food with their bare hands?
What facilities exist for reducing the handling of food i.e. tongs, food slicers etc.?
Are there arrangements for staff screening on joining the organization, and on returning from holidays abroad?
What are the reporting procedures for staff food handlers suffering from gastro-intestinal illnesses?

Do staff avoid wearing rings, watches, earrings, etc. whilst handling open high risk foods?

14 PROTECTIVE CLOTHING

Is the standard of cleanliness and the provision of protective clothing satisfactory and appropriate?
Are the head coverings suitable to prevent hair falling into food?
Is the storage for outdoor clothing adequate?

15 STAFF TRAINING

Do staff receive training in food hygiene?
What level of training is being given to staff?
What management controls exist to promote and enforce hygiene standards?
What is the management attitude to staff training?

Accident Book

'An Accident Book should be kept on the premises readily accessible at all reasonable times to any employed earner and any person bonafide acting on his behalf.'

An accident book can be purchased from Her Majesty's Stationery Office and all premises are obliged to keep one under Social Security Act 1975 'where ten or more persons are normally employed at the same time' but if there are less than ten employees, still keep some sort of record of the report of an accident, especially if an 'injury results in the person injured being admitted into hospital as an in-patient for more than twenty-four hours.'

Index